Mayo Clinic on Headache

Jerry W. Swanson, M.D.

Editor in Chief

Mayo Clinic
Rochester, Minnesota

Mayo Clinic on Headache is a practical guide for the millions of individuals who get headaches, either occasionally or frequently. Much of the information comes directly from the experience of physicians, nurses, research scientists and other health care professionals at Mayo Clinic. This book supplements the advice of your personal physician, whom you should consult for individual medical problems. *Mayo Clinic on Headache* does not endorse any company or product. MAYO, MAYO CLINIC, MAYO CLINIC HEALTH INFORMATION and the Mayo triple-shield logo are marks of Mayo Foundation for Medical Education and Research.

Published by Mayo Clinic Health Information, Rochester, Minn. Distributed to the book trade by Kensington Publishing Corporation, New York, N.Y.

Photo credits: Cover photos and the photos on pages 1, 23, 41, 43, 63, 69, 72, 75, 77, 83, 90, 124, 143, 161, 172, 182 and C3 are from PhotoDisc®.

Library of Congress Catalog Card Number: 2004105801

ISBN 1-893005-35-6

Printed in the United States of America

First Edition

1 2 3 4 5 6 7 8 9 10

About headache

Virtually everyone experiences a headache at some time during his or her life. But many don't realize just how different that experience can be from one individual to the next. Head pain can range from mild to severe, and last several seconds or several hours. Attacks can occur once a year or multiple times in one day. A headache may not interfere in the daily routine or it may be disabling and shut down all activities. Along with this broad range of experiences, people must confront many social misperceptions about headaches and their impact on individuals' lives.

The fourteenth book in Mayo's On Health series, *Mayo Clinic on Headache* provides you with clear explanations of different types of headache and the best strategies for treating and managing these conditions. The text is supplemented by drawings and photographs in an eight-page color section. A glossary and listing of additional resources are included at the back of the book.

About Mayo Clinic

Mayo Clinic evolved from the frontier practice of Dr. William Worrall Mayo and the partnership of his two sons, William J. and Charles H. Mayo, in the early 1900s. Pressed by the demands of their busy practice in Rochester, Minn., the Mayo brothers invited other physicians to join them, pioneering the private group practice of medicine. Today, with more than 2,000 physicians and scientists at its three major locations in Rochester, Minn., Jacksonville, Fla., and Scottsdale, Ariz., Mayo Clinic is dedicated to providing comprehensive diagnoses, accurate answers and effective treatments.

With this depth of medical knowledge, experience and expertise, Mayo Clinic occupies an unparalleled position as a health information resource. Since 1983, Mayo Clinic has published reliable health information for millions of consumers through award-winning newsletters, books and online services. Revenue from the publishing activities supports Mayo Clinic programs, including medical education and research.

Editorial staff

Editor in Chief
Jerry W. Swanson, M.D.

Managing Editor
Kevin Kaufman

Copy Editor
Judy Duguid

Proofreading
Miranda Attlesey
Mary Duerson
Louise Filipic
Donna Hanson

Contributing Writers
Lee Engfer
Julie Freeman
Rachel Bartony
Jennifer Jacobson
Amy Michenfelder

Editorial Research
Anthony Cook
Dana Gerberi
Deirdre Herman
Michelle Hewlett
Stephen Johnson

Creative Director
Daniel Brevick

Art Director
Brian Fyffe

Illustration and Photography
Kent McDaniel
Christopher Srnka

Medical Illustration
Michael King

Indexing
Larry Harrison

Contributing editors and reviewers

J. D. Bartleson, M.D.
David Black, M.D.
Christopher Boes, M.D.
David Capobianco, M.D.
F. Michael Cutrer, M.D.
David Dodick, M.D.
Eric Eross, D.O.

Christopher Frye
Karina Huerter, P.A.-C.
Susan Lewis, R.N.
Linda Linbo, R.N.
Kenneth Mack, M.D.
Robert Rogers, P.A.-C.
Christopher Sletten, Ph.D.

Preface

Headache is nearly a universal human phenomenon. In fact, statistically it's abnormal for an individual not to experience a headache at times. On the other hand, there's seemingly endless variation in the causes and symptoms of different headaches. For instance, there are headache disorders that are the result of a serious underlying condition such as a brain tumor, meningitis, or hydrocephalus. There also are headaches that are classified primary headache disorders, such as migraine, with no known underlying cause. Even the impact of a specific type of headache can vary greatly from individual to individual. For example, some individuals may have occasional migraine attacks yet they remain productive and still able to go about their lives. For other individuals, the attacks may be frequent, severe and disabling. Because of the heterogeneity of headache problems, it's sometimes difficult for health care professionals, as well as the general public, to appreciate the disruption that some individuals experience with their headaches.

There have been major advances in the understanding of various headache disorders in recent years. This book, based on the latest knowledge, details the steps to appropriate diagnosis and treatment of headaches. It offers practical guidance that will help individuals understand their headaches and direct them to the sources of support that are available. This information can greatly assist individuals who experience headaches, as well as their family and friends.

Headache specialists in the Department of Neurology at Mayo Clinic facilities in Rochester, Minnesota, Jacksonville, Florida and Scottsdale, Arizona have reviewed the content of this book for accuracy. The result, we hope, is a concise, understandable and practical resource that will help individuals to successfully manage their headaches.

Jerry W. Swanson, M.D.
Editor in Chief

Contents

Part 2: Migraine

Part 3: Other types of headache

Part 4: Special issues

Part 1

Understanding headache

Chapter 1

Introduction to headache

After dropping the children off at school and fighting morning traffic, you arrive at the office to find your inbox full and your schedule overloaded. You have a report due by 10 a.m. and you haven't even had your morning coffee. A ringing phone and office clutter only add to the mounting stress. Already your head is hurting, but you continue about your tasks. The dull pain lasts for several hours until the morning rush subsides.

The above scenario describes the classic headache that's commonly triggered by stress. But this description doesn't apply to all headaches. In fact, one of the most remarkable aspects of headache is the sheer variety. There's such variation in the nature of pain, the frequency and duration of attacks, and the presence of other symptoms, that it's difficult to characterize everyone's experience. The unifying feature is that everyone's head hurts.

Here's a scenario involving a different kind of headache: You stop by the library to make photocopies. The book you're using requires the photocopier lid to be left open for the pages to lie flat. You make the mistake of looking down as copies are being made, and bright lights flash in your eyes. A throbbing headache develops minutes later. Your eyesight becomes blurred and you feel nauseated. You return home and lie quietly in a darkened room. This is a headache that has repeated itself for years.

Another kind of headache is described in this scenario: You go to bed at your regular time but awaken around 1:30 a.m. with an excruciating headache. Searing pain bores into your skull, focused behind one eye. The eye begins to water, and the nostril on that same side becomes stuffy. Unable to remain lying down, you pace back and forth and wait for the pain to subside, which usually takes about an hour. But you know that this attack signals the beginning of a new round of headaches. After being relatively pain-free for months, similar headaches will continue to strike several times each day over a period of weeks.

All these scenarios depict different versions of the same condition — a headache. Each scenario describes a different kind of head pain that develops under different circumstances and has a different impact on your ability to function in daily life. With so many variations, the question is what exactly is a headache?

Defining headache

The word *headache* can describe almost any type of pain felt in the head. And the pain may be in any part of the head — not only in the areas of the temple and forehead that people normally associate with headache, but also at the back of the head and in the lower face. Another word for headache is *cephalalgia* (sef-uh-LAL-juh), originating from an ancient Greek word meaning "head pain."

A headache is a medical problem, just as heart disease and high blood pressure are. The pain may be sharp, dull, constant, intermittent, aching or throbbing. It may last for seconds, minutes, hours or days. You may experience the pain on just one side of your head or on both. You may have a headache attack with features of more than one type of headache, or you may experience different headaches at different times. Sometimes, it's simply hard to describe your symptoms or to pinpoint when the pain started.

Why do headaches occur? Scientists don't have all the answers yet, although a medical understanding of headaches and the treatment options for them are ever improving and expanding. It's reasonable to believe that headaches result from interactions between your brain, nerves and blood vessels. But these interactions are extremely complex. Some headaches develop for obvious reasons, such as the result of a blow to the head. Often, headaches start without obvious injury or other clear source of the pain.

Why do some people get headaches more often than others? You simply may be prone to headaches because of your genetic makeup and brain chemistry. In the case of migraine, the problem can be hereditary. Children whose parents have migraines are more likely to also have migraines. Lifestyle may also be a factor. Some headaches are related to being stressed out, feeling overworked, not getting enough sleep or skipping meals.

A common ailment

Almost everyone has experienced a headache at one time or another. Some headaches are only mildly painful, while others are severe. No matter what kind of headache you have, it's likely you'd rather be without it.

In the United States, headache makes the top-20 list of the most common complaint heard by family practitioners. One study found that approximately 95 percent of women and 91 percent of men experienced at least one headache during a 12-month period. Most headaches reported in the study were resolved with self-care, as only 18 percent of female participants and 15 percent of male participants consulted a doctor.

Furthermore, the number of people who suffer from chronic, or recurring, headaches is astounding — in the United States, more than 45 million Americans. In fact, the number of Americans who have chronic headaches far exceeds the combined total of those Americans who have diabetes, asthma and coronary heart disease. And of those 45 million, more than half — 28 million people — experience the headache known as migraine.

Unfortunately, children, even infants, can experience headache as easily as adults. Migraine has been diagnosed in children as young as age 3. In addition, it's estimated that between 7 percent and 18 percent of children, boys and girls alike, have migraine.

By and large, headache is more prevalent during early adulthood and becomes less common after middle age. For instance, migraine is most common in people between the ages of 25 and 55 — a time when most of us are in our peak work years. That's why headache has such an impact on the American workforce.

Women experience headache, particularly migraine, more often than men do. This may be, in part, because migraine can be influenced by changes in hormone levels, such as what occurs during a woman's menstrual cycle or during her pregnancy. But men get migraine, too, and not all women develop migraine when they have their periods. Most women who get migraine experience them throughout the month, even at times when their hormones are not fluctuating greatly.

Fortunately, most people have mild or infrequent headaches and don't need to see a doctor about them. Over-the-counter pain relievers and simple preventive steps help manage the problem. However, headache is a serious concern for some. These people experience severe, incapacitating headaches that aren't relieved by over-the-counter medications. Or they have frequent — even perhaps daily — headaches that take a heavy toll on their abilities to function physically and emotionally.

A visit to the doctor may be in order under these circumstances. Your doctor may prescribe more effective pain relievers and other medications to treat your headache. In addition, your doctor may recommend simple lifestyle changes to prevent headache.

Myths about headache

Misperceptions about headache abound. For example, there's a tendency among many people to think that all headaches are the same. And there's a perception that rising levels of stress always cause headaches. This correlation is certainly true for some people — and equally untrue for others. That's where the confusion arises. Stress may very well trigger a headache in someone susceptible to migraine. On the other hand, in a person who's not susceptible to getting a headache, it's unlikely that stress will cause one.

Advertising perpetuates common misperceptions about headache in today's society. In many advertisements, for example, headache remedies are portrayed as miracle drugs that relieve the toughest head pain in minutes. In reality, not all headaches can be wiped away by taking a pill. Medications are just one part, although a vital part, of most treatment programs. Very often, effective nondrug therapies are necessary in combination with drugs.

Not only do loved ones, friends and coworkers frequently misperceive the impact that headache can have on someone. Often, the individuals themselves who have headaches end up believing they're to blame for the problem. This misperception may prevent some people from seeking help for their headaches.

The good news is that separating fact from myth can help you seek out the best available treatment for your headache. Here are a few common myths associated with headache, along with corresponding facts that may counter these misperceptions:

Headaches are all in your head. A headache isn't something that you imagine or cause to happen. A headache is a medical condition caused by physiological events. As with other chronic conditions, recurring headaches require medical care and self-care measures in order to manage them. They're not just a complaint from someone who's hysterical or a hypochondriac.

Headaches mean there's something emotionally wrong. Chronic headaches aren't a sign of psychological problems. They're a biological disorder. While some people with mental health problems get headaches, the headaches aren't necessarily a result of these problems. And while people enduring the pain of a throbbing headache may become irritable or moody, that doesn't mean they have a mental disorder. Unfortunately, some people, particularly men, are reluctant to see a doctor about headache because they don't wish to appear unable to handle the problem on their own.

People who complain about headaches can't handle pain. No scientific evidence suggests that people with severe migraines, for example, are more sensitive to pain than those who don't have migraines. The fact that many people are able to carry on with everyday activities despite migraines demonstrates how resilient they are. Perhaps, this particular myth is pervasive in society at large because many people mistakenly refer to all headaches as migraines. Actually, the pain of a migraine is more intense than many other kinds of headache pain. A believer of this myth may have never experienced pain of that severity.

Headaches are an excuse to avoid obligations. In television comedies, a woman wishing to avoid intimacy with her husband may use the familiar line: "Not tonight, honey. I have a headache." In reality, a severe headache is not just a convenient excuse. People who experience chronic headaches have a legitimate reason to miss household obligations, work or social activities. The fact that a few people use headaches as an excuse to get out of doing something doesn't mean that everyone with a headache is taking advantage of his or her condition.

Headaches aren't anything serious. Fortunately, the vast majority of headaches are not the result of serious underlying disorders. But there are certain warning signs of headache that you should be aware of. If you experience a sudden, severe headache that is unlike any you've ever had before or headaches that continue to worsen over time, you should see a doctor promptly for an evaluation. Also see a doctor immediately if you experience a headache associated with high fever or stiff neck. Other headache warning signs are discussed in Chapter 3.

Recurrent headaches are something you live with. If headaches are affecting your ability to function in daily life, you should see your doctor. Don't let apprehension or indecision stop you from getting help. Often, proper medical attention and lifestyle changes will allow you to have the active, involved, independent lifestyle that you choose to lead.

Social impact of headache

Anyone who has ever had headaches knows they cause pain. Many people also are aware of other signs and symptoms, such as nausea, that accompany some headaches. What often goes unrecognized or unacknowledged, however, is how disruptive headaches can be on day-to-day living. The disruption extends well beyond the times when your head actually hurts. Studies show that headache upsets family life, leisure time and career path more than many other chronic disorders.

People with migraine, for example, may find the pain so severe that they miss work, school and social engagements whenever attacks occur. Nausea and vomiting that accompany the attacks may make it impossible even to function at home. Sensitivity to light and sound may force someone to retire to a quiet, dark room and lie down until the pain has passed. If the migraine attacks are frequent, this very quickly adds up to a lot of missed days of work or school, a significant reduction of social interaction, and the inability to pursue personal goals or favorite pastimes.

In fact, headache is one of the most common reasons why people miss work. Severe head pain may cause a person, unwillingly, to leave work suddenly, curtail meetings or simply stay at home. On average, people with migraine miss over 4 workdays per year. And this fact doesn't take into account the loss of productivity among workers with headaches who, although struggling to stay on task, must remain or choose to remain at their jobs.

Even when headaches aren't present, there are emotional pressures to deal with. One difficult aspect of recurring headaches is that they make you feel as though you've lost self-control. Headache attacks can be unpredictable and arrive at moments when you need to be at your best. This makes it hard to plan ahead or organize your schedule with assurance. You may feel sensitive to the scrutiny of others, whether real or imagined, for claiming to have a condition with so few visible signs. Because you've canceled plans in the past or are hesitant to participate in some activities, you may feel socially isolated.

Studies have found that migraine raises a person's risk of developing depression. There appears to be underlying biological causes for both migraine and depression that have things in common. Also, it's understandable that people who experience severe headaches with a disruption of family, work and social activities often become depressed. They must continually stop what they're doing, change plans and explain their actions to others when they have headaches or as they attempt to avoid them.

Headache may cause an individual plenty of discomfort and insecurity. But headache also takes its toll on employers. In fact, headache is listed among the top five most costly health conditions to U.S. employers. The National Headache Foundation estimates that American businesses lose approximately $50 billion a year due to absenteeism and medical expenses caused by headache. People with chronic, severe headaches may lose their jobs or face prejudices in the workplace because of their condition.

This makes headache more than just a nuisance. The condition has a profound, wide-ranging impact both on individuals and on society at large.

Taking action

Many people rely only on self-medication for headaches, usually with over-the-counter pain relievers, even when these remedies aren't effective. Others try to hide or ignore the fact that they have the condition. But if headaches are disrupting your work or social life, it's time to consider other actions. While headaches can't always be prevented, the symptoms usually can be managed with proper medical treatment.

If you're experiencing headaches and it's not clear what's causing them or what can make them better, you should consider consulting your doctor. The problem can be diagnosed, and you and your doctor can work together to find an effective treatment. As will be discussed in later chapters, there are a variety of effective and readily available drug and nondrug options.

Not getting medical advice for recurring headaches or severe headache pain may end up being more costly than a visit to the doctor. The time and money you spend each year to relieve disabling pain may be greater than the time and money you would have spent on a physician-recommended treatment.

Chapter 2

Types of headaches

Headaches come in all shapes and sizes. Chapter 1 described how pain can vary from mild to intense, from dull to stabbing. Attacks can be occasional, but some people have headaches every day. In addition, symptoms such as nausea may or may not accompany the head pain.

How, then, do physicians and researchers know one type of headache from another? Drawing on years of shared experience in medical practice and research, specialists have identified headache variables and have organized different types of headaches in a comprehensive system. This classification is the likely basis for a clinical diagnosis you may receive from your doctor.

Classifying headaches

The International Headache Society (IHS) led an effort to identify and define the different types of headaches in the 1980s. The IHS assembled headache specialists from around the world to help with the creation of the International Classification of Headache Disorders. A revised classification was published in 2003. This system is the gold standard for describing headaches and is used in research as well as some situations in clinical practice.

The classification divides all headaches into 14 major groups. Groups 1 through 4 are known as primary headaches, based on their signs and symptoms. Groups 5 through 12 are known as secondary headaches, grouped according to their different causes. Groups 13 and 14 include forms of neuralgias — pain associated with nerve fibers — and facial pain as well as rare forms of headaches not associated with the preceding groups.

Each headache group is subdivided into types and subtypes. A description accompanies each headache entry along with a list of criteria, in precise and unambiguous language, required for a physician to make the diagnosis. Entries at each level of the classification system — group, type and subtype — are designated with a number, or code, that indicates where each distinct headache fits within the system. In this way, the many different types of headaches are clearly identified.

How is this headache classification system used? It provides common terminology that doctors and researchers around the world can use, regardless of what their specialization is, where they work or what language they speak. The list of specific criteria that accompany each headache entry makes diagnoses more uniform and universally understood. Many treatments for headache have been developed on the basis of this classification. Furthermore, the system can assist you in understanding your headache and describing the signs and symptoms you may be experiencing.

Primary headaches

Primary headaches are headaches that aren't caused by underlying health problems. There's no clear source for the pain. The vast majority of headaches that people experience are primary headaches. Although their causes are poorly understood, a tendency to develop some of them seems to be inherited. The four major groups of primary headaches are:

Migraine. Moderate to severe pain characterizes a migraine. Around 60 percent of people with migraine (sometimes called migraineurs) have pain only on one side of the head, while the other 40 percent experience pain on both sides. A migraine in an adult may last from four to 72 hours, but the frequency of attacks

**Major headache groups according to
the International Classification of Headache Disorders**

Primary headache disorders
1. Migraine
2. Tension-type headache
3. Cluster headache and other trigeminal autonomic cephalalgias
4. Other primary headaches

Secondary headache disorders
5. Headache attributed to head and neck trauma
6. Headache attributed to cranial or cervical vascular disorder
7. Headache attributed to nonvascular intracranial disorder
8. Headache attributed to a substance or its withdrawal
9. Headache attributed to infection
10. Headache attributed to disorder of homeostasis
11. Headache or facial pain attributed to disorder of cranium, neck, eyes, ears, nose, sinuses, teeth, mouth, or other facial or cranial structures
12. Headache attributed to psychiatric disorder

Cranial neuralgias, primary facial pain and other headaches
13. Cranial neuralgias and central causes of facial pain
14. Other headaches, cranial neuralgia, and central or primary facial pain

varies from individual to individual. Some people have an attack twice a year, others several times in a month.

The head pain is often part of what's known as a multisymptom complex, because other symptoms may also be present during the migraine, such as nausea and sensitivity to light and sound. Some migraineurs have an aura preceding the attack. Aura is a variety of sensations that includes blind spots and bright flashes in the field of vision, dizziness, and numbness or tingling. More details on migraine are provided in Chapters 4 through 7.

Tension-type headache. This headache is the most common form of primary headache. It usually produces a dull pain, tightness, or band of pressure in your forehead and scalp or at the back of your neck. A tension-type headache may occur occasionally or almost daily. A single attack can last from 30 minutes to an entire week. See Chapter 8 for more about this headache. If attacks occur more than 15 days a month for at least three months, it's considered a chronic form. Some people have headaches with features of both migraine and tension-type headache. These are sometimes called combination headaches or mixed tension migraine.

Cluster headache. This primary headache is characterized by severe, boring pain in and around one eye or on one side of your head. A series of these intense headaches occurs in clusters of attacks — hence the name. Cluster headache can occur daily for days, weeks or months at a time and then disappear completely for months or even years. The pain typically intensifies within five to 10 minutes to a peak that may last from 15 minutes to three hours. More details on cluster headache are provided in Chapter 10.

Other primary headaches. This group consists of various primary headaches that don't fit into the three preceding groups. Many of these are short-lasting headaches with characteristic signs and symptoms. Examples include headaches caused by coughing or sneezing or by prolonged physical exercise. Other types include the aptly named thunderclap headache as well as the hypnic headache, which affects primarily older adults.

Secondary headaches

Headaches that are a symptom of another disease or condition are called secondary headaches. Head pain is not the primary problem, but rather is a result of the primary problem. Secondary head-aches are divided into eight major groups, according to the different causes. The groups are listed below — although keep in mind that there are hundreds of causes of secondary headaches.

- **Head or neck trauma.** Headaches can be the result of mild to moderate impact or injury to the head or neck, even if there has been no loss of consciousness. Whiplash following a car accident is a typical example of this kind of trauma.
- **Vascular disorders within the cranium.** Blood vessel disorders that may cause headaches include stroke, high blood

pressure, inflammation of the arteries or a ruptured blood vessel in the membranes between the skull and brain.

- **Nonvascular disorders within the cranium.** Headaches may result from abnormal pressure on brain tissue caused by tumors or an increase in the pressure of your cerebrospinal fluid (the fluid that surrounds and cushions your brain).
- **Abuse of substances such as drugs, tobacco or alcohol.** The addictive qualities of tobacco and alcohol are well known. Sometimes people who overuse pain relievers for headaches may in fact be getting headaches from their pain relief medication (rebound headaches).
- **Viral and bacterial infections.** Many intracranial infections, including meningitis and encephalitis, can cause headaches. In fact, headache is often one of the earliest symptoms. With systemic infections, which affect the body generally, headache is often present but less conspicuous. A common example of systemic infection is influenza (flu).
- **Disorders of homeostasis.** Certain processes keep physiological conditions, such as body temperature, relatively stable, or in a state of homeostasis. Disorders that disrupt these processes are known to cause headaches. They include problems with the thyroid gland, which helps regulate growth, and oxygen deficiency brought on by high altitudes.
- **Disorders of your neck, eyes, ears, nose, sinuses, teeth or other cranial structures.** Headaches may accompany but are not necessarily the direct result of a disorder of certain cranial structures. One example would be headaches attributed to temporomandibular joint disease, when the joint that hinges the lower jaw to your skull malfunctions.
- **Psychiatric disorders.** Headaches, although rarely, may be associated with psychiatric conditions such as somatization disorder, in which a mental state is converted into a bodily symptom, and delusional disorder, involving firmly held beliefs that have no basis in reality.

Usually, secondary headaches go away when the primary problems are resolved. Treatment varies depending on the type of underlying health condition you have.

Cranial neuralgias, other facial pain and other headaches

Pain in the neck or on the face may result from nerves being subjected to pressure or physical injury, being exposed to cold, or other forms of irritation. There are 12 pairs of cranial nerves originating from your brain and extending to your face, neck and other parts of your body. The trigeminal nerve, the fifth of these 12 nerve pairs, carries sensations from your face to your brain. Disruption of the normal function of the trigeminal nerve can cause a painful condition known as trigeminal neuralgia (see Chapter 11).

The headache classification system designates the last group as the place to add descriptions of what may be new, unique headache types. It also includes unspecified headaches that have been reported but about which there's simply not enough information to be able to classify them.

What is pain?

Pain is a universal experience, and headache pain is one of the most common complaints. But how your mind and body perceive pain is a question that scientists are still pondering.

In general, pain appears to start with a series of exchanges within your nervous system. Your nervous system is composed of nerve cells that transmit and receive messages in the form of electric currents and chemical interactions. It's through this intricate network of cells that your brain communicates with the rest of your body.

The two main components of your nervous system are your central nervous system, which includes your brain and spinal cord, and your peripheral nervous system, comprised of nerves that extend throughout the rest of your body. Some peripheral nerves have special nerve endings, called nociceptors (no-sih-SEP-turs), that can sense an unpleasant stimulus, such as a cut, burn or inflammation. When nociceptors detect a harmful stimulus, they relay their pain messages in the form of electric impulses through the peripheral nerve network to your spinal cord and brain.

When pain messages reach your brain, they arrive at the thalamus, a clearinghouse for information that needs to be relayed to

Acute, chronic and episodic pain

The terms *acute, chronic* and *episodic* are often used to distinguish one headache type from another. One of these terms may designate your specific condition. Although you may have a general idea of what they mean, it's worthwhile taking the time to understand each term with regard to headache.

Acute. Describes a headache that is severe and lasts a short time. The onset may be sudden. Many secondary headaches are acute conditions.

Chronic. Describes a headache that occurs frequently over a long period of time. For example, if tension-type headaches occur more than 15 days in a month for at least three months, the condition is designated chronic. For some types of chronic headaches, the occurrences get progressively worse.

Episodic. Describes a headache that is a separate event but still forming part of a larger series. For example, if tension-type headaches occur on 15 days or fewer in a month — meaning each headache has a definite beginning and ending separated by discrete periods of time — the condition is designated an episodic headache.

It's important to note that the criteria for these terms may change from one headache type to another. For example, cluster headache is chronic if the attacks occur daily for more than a year with pain-free periods lasting less than one month. Cluster headache is episodic if the attacks occur daily for a period of one week to one year, separated by pain-free periods lasting one month or more.

Also note that acute headaches can have episodic characteristics. For example, acute migraine occurs at variable intervals, whether once a year or several times a month.

other parts of the brain. The thalamus interprets the pain messages and forwards them to three specialized regions dealing with physical sensation (somatosensory cortex), emotions (limbic system) and thinking (frontal cortex). Your awareness of pain is therefore a complex experience of sensing, feeling and thinking.

What causes headache pain?

It's a fact that brain tissue can't ache because there are no nerves in brain tissue. Brain operations have been performed when people are conscious and they reported no pain. Only certain structures in your head are pain-sensitive. Some of these structures are your eyes, your teeth, your sinuses, the large blood vessels, the membranes that envelop your brain, the membranes that cover bones, and the nerves associated with your cranium and spinal cord.

So just what is happening when your head hurts? The causes of many primary headaches are unclear, but research on migraine provides some rudimentary answers for this type of headache. Studies suggest that migraine is associated with changes in the levels of certain brain chemicals called neurotransmitters. One of these chemicals is serotonin, which regulates pain messages to the brain (see page C2 of the Color Section). The level of endorphins — natural painkillers — also may change.

Such alterations in your brain chemistry appear to activate the trigeminal nerve — one of the 12 cranial nerve pairs and a major pain pathway to your brain — causing the blood vessels in your head to dilate and become inflamed. The special nerve endings that respond to pain (nociceptors) within these blood vessels alert the brain, officially registering a migraine.

Genetic predisposition

Most scientists agree that primary headaches have a genetic component. In other words, if you have problems with headache, you've probably inherited a body chemistry from your parents that makes you susceptible to headache. With a genetic predisposition, certain factors that may not bother others — such as stress, hormones or red wine — may bring on a headache in you.

A genetic link to headache is revealed in a rare form of migraine called familial hemiplegic migraine (FHM). FHM is characterized by a variety of signs and symptoms that may include aura, temporary paralysis on one side of the body (hemiplegia), coma, eye

Theories about migraine

Migraine is the most studied of all headaches, and there are a number of competing theories about what may actually cause them. Some of these theories have become outdated. For example, for years many scientists believed that migraine was caused by a disturbance in the large blood vessels of your head. Over time, this theory was found to be too simplistic for explaining the complexities of these headaches.

Other theories are just forming. Here are two examples:

Hyperexcitability of the brain. This theory assumes that a genetic defect causes an abnormal release of neurotransmitters in your brain. This leads to what's called a state of hyperexcitability in your brain and an abnormal response to one or more stimulating factors.

Migraine generator. Another current theory involves the mechanisms in your brain that control pain and blood flow. These mechanisms may be triggered to malfunction, causing nerve cells to become hypersensitive and creating what one scientist calls a "nerve storm" in your head. As such, your brain might be considered a migraine generator that's activated by normal input from the environment, such as sounds or smells.

problems and mental impairment. In approximately half the families with FHM, the condition has been linked to a genetic defect on chromosome 19 — one of the 23 groups of DNA contained in almost every human cell. In another 15 percent of FHM families, the condition is linked to a mutation on chromosome 1. A genetic mutation among the remaining families still has not been detected. But these findings may provide clues to the genetic elements involved in other types of migraine as well as FHM.

The genetic makeup that underlies headache isn't just a simple issue involving one defective gene. Scientists are convinced that multiple genes are involved. Furthermore, they know that genes aren't the whole story. Environmental factors also contribute to the development of headache. It's estimated that genes are involved in approximately 40 percent to 50 percent of headache disorders.

Headache triggers

Whatever the mechanism in your brain that's involved in headache, something in the environment often triggers it. Triggers can be almost anything. Migraine can be triggered by certain foods, changes in weather or sleeping patterns, exposure to bright lights or unusual odors, skipping a meal, drinking alcohol, having sex, and other possibilities. For women who have migraine, the trigger often appears to be a drop in levels of the hormone estrogen. Tension-type headache may be triggered by poor posture, working in awkward positions, stress, depression and anxiety.

Although a propensity for headache may be inherited by several members of a family, the headache triggers seem to be unique to each person. For example, alcohol may trigger a migraine in your mother but not in you. Your migraine may be brought on by certain smells that don't affect your mother. This happens because each person, even within the same family, becomes sensitive to different environmental factors. See Chapter 4 for more detail on different types of migraine triggers.

Discovering what triggers your headaches is often helpful in managing your condition. But you should be aware that identifying a trigger is not as straightforward as it sounds. Some people find it useful to keep a headache diary, which, over time, may reveal patterns and factors that seem to be causing headache.

Chapter 3

Diagnosing headache

If you're like most people, you've experienced at least a mild headache from time to time. And, like most people, you probably don't run to your doctor with concerns about minor head pain that passes within a short time. Very often, mild headache can be relieved simply with over-the-counter pain relievers or a few moments of relaxation.

For millions of Americans, though, headaches are a medical problem. Over-the-counter medications don't provide sufficient relief. But even when headache pain is severe or disabling, many people hesitate to admit that they're bothered by headaches. After all, the old belief that headaches are purely psychological is a difficult one to put to rest.

Warning signs

The term *headache*, as discussed previously, describes almost any pain that occurs in the head. There are many types of headaches because there are so many possible causes of head pain.

There are two common reasons why people feel they should seek medical care for headache. Either they fear the headache is caused by a serious underlying condition, or the headache prevents them from functioning normally and participating in work, family and social activities. For either reason, seeing the doctor is the correct course of action.

Fortunately, most headaches, although painful and sometimes disabling, aren't life-threatening and are treatable. A doctor's diagnosis is an essential first step for treatment to begin.

There are certain developments that indicate potential problems if you have recurrent headaches. Consider contacting your doctor if you notice any of the following patterns forming:

- You usually have three or more headaches per week.
- You must take a pain reliever every day or almost daily for your headaches.
- You feel that you need more than the recommended doses of over-the-counter medications to relieve pain.

Some headache symptoms may signal the need for more prompt medical attention. You should plan to see your doctor if you experience any of the following:

- Your headaches keep getting worse and won't go away.
- The severity, duration and frequency of your headaches have increased noticeably.
- You develop persistent headaches after being relatively headache-free in the past.
- Your headaches are triggered by coughing, bending, physical exertion or sexual activity.
- Your headaches started following trauma to your head.
- Your headaches began after age 50.

Some types of head pain may warn of more sinister disorders and call for prompt medical care (see sidebar "Headache alarms"). Rare but serious causes of headache include brain tumor, stroke, aneurysm, temporal arteritis, meningitis and encephalitis.

Initial doctor visit

Your doctor likely will begin the office visit with an interview, asking questions and listening to your description of head pain and other symptoms. Often, a detailed question-and-answer session can

Headache alarms

Any of the following signs and symptoms should alert you that a serious medical condition may be the cause of your headache and you should seek immediate medical attention. If you can't see your doctor right away, you should go to the hospital emergency room if:

- You experience a severe headache for the first time.
- Your headache is the worst you've ever had.
- Your headache comes on suddenly and severely — a so-called thunderclap headache.
- You experience numbness, lack of coordination, double vision, slurred speech or weakness on one side of your body.
- You experience fever, stiff neck, sore muscles or joints, vision loss, or jaw pain when you chew.
- You experience confusion or drowsiness with a headache.
- Persistent or severe vomiting or seizures accompany a headache.
- You have cancer, HIV (the virus that causes AIDS) or another serious condition and develop new headaches.

produce enough information about your headache for the doctor to form at least an initial diagnosis.

When evaluating someone's headache, the doctor's first task is either to identify or to exclude any underlying cause of the pain that may require treatment. If it appears that no underlying condition is to blame for your headache, the doctor will try to determine what type of primary headache you're experiencing, which is not always an easy task.

The doctor also will obtain a medical history and may perform a physical examination of your head, eyes, ears, nose and throat. A neurological examination may be undertaken. If the doctor suspects that an underlying condition may be causing your headache, you may be screened with laboratory tests such as blood or urine tests. Your doctor also may suggest that you undergo a brain scan to look for the cause of your headache.

The interview

When evaluating a headache, the doctor looks for patterns that are characteristic of a specific type of headache. The doctor's interview may be like playing the childhood game, twenty questions:

- Do you seem to have more than one type of headache? For example, do you have a mild, aching pain that develops daily but also have occasional attacks of severe, throbbing pain? For each type of headache, you'll need to answer a similar set of questions.
- When did the headaches start? How old were you when they began? Did they begin following an illness, trauma or other specific event, or did they start spontaneously?
- How often do the headaches occur? If they occur frequently, do attacks happen several times daily? Is the pain continuous, or do painful episodes occur intermittently?
- Where is the pain located? For example, is the pain on your forehead or around one eye? Is it on one side only? If the pain is on just one side, is it always on the same side?
- How would you describe the pain? Is it throbbing? Do you experience a dull, steady ache or a band-like sensation of pressure? Does the character of the pain change over time? How bad would you rate your pain on a scale of 1 to 10?
- How long do your headaches typically last? What's the shortest or longest amount of time?
- When do you develop headaches? Do they begin suddenly or gradually? Do they strike at the same time of day? Do your headaches awaken you from sleep? Do they occur upon waking in the morning? Are your headaches affected by weekends, travel or other breaks in your routine?
- Do other symptoms accompany the pain? Do you get warning signs before the headaches begin? What happens during the headaches? What symptoms do you have right now?
- Are there any factors that may trigger or aggravate the pain? Have you been bothered by stress, changes in sleep patterns, hunger, changes in the weather, or physical activity? Are your headaches worse when you're lying down or standing up? Are they aggravated by straining or lifting? Do they occur at a spe-

Describing pain

You know for sure that your head hurts, but what does the pain feel like? Is it constant or intermittent? Is it aching and dull or sharp and stabbing? Where on your head is the pain located — focused at one spot or generalized across your forehead and temples? Is the pain disabling, or are you still able to carry on with daily activities? Different kinds of pain characterize different kinds of headaches. Describing your pain clearly can help your doctor identify the type of headache you have.

Discussing the exact nature of your pain may seem difficult when you first try it. Here's a list of words and phrases that may help you:

Shooting	Stabbing	Throbbing
Pulsating	Aching	Hammering
Heavy	Stinging	Head in a vise
Pins and needles	Feeling of pressure	Electric, shock-like

Your doctor may ask you to rank your headache pain on a scale from 1 to 10, with 1 being mild pain and 10 being severe pain. In addition, it's important to know how disabling your headaches are. How often do they cause you to miss work or social functions? Do they interfere with your relationships or your family life? Ranking the severity of your pain and identifying the level of disability it causes can influence the diagnosis and treatment.

cific time related to your menstrual period? Have they begun or worsened during pregnancy?

- What helps your headaches? What medications have you tried to relieve pain? What doses were used? Which medication seemed to work best? Were any nondrug therapies or home treatments effective?

Your doctor likely will ask about your workday, family life and sleep habits. For example, are any areas of your life a source of great stress? Have you recently experienced a marriage, divorce, new job, retirement or death in the family? How many days from work or school do you miss each month? What activities are you unable to participate in when a headache strikes? Are you able to get enough rest and relaxation?

Try to be as precise and complete in your answers as possible. Let your doctor know whether you feel discouraged, and try to communicate what you would like him or her to do to help you manage the pain. The better you can describe your headache, the easier it will be for your doctor to reach an accurate diagnosis and gauge what type of treatment would be most appropriate.

Before seeing your doctor, you may want to write down any questions you wish to discuss during the visit. You also should list all the medications you take, including over-the-counter drugs, prescription drugs and any vitamins or supplements. Your doctor likely will ask for such a list. A history of prior headache treatments is necessary for the evaluation.

Your doctor may ask you to track your headaches in a diary or calendar, either before or after the first office visit. A headache diary helps you record information about your headaches over a period of time. You're typically asked to log details about each attack, including the environment in which the attacks took place, possible headache triggers and what helped relieve the pain.

Your medical history
Your medical history is a tool that your doctor depends on to evaluate a headache. This history includes previous test results — for example, tests to screen for blood pressure or vision — and names of all the medications or supplements that you're currently taking. Your doctor will also require basic information about any medical condition and serious injury that you're being treated for or you've experienced in the past. The information you provide should give the doctor a comprehensive picture of your overall health, as well as any associated problems that could influence treatment.

Your doctor also may inquire about your family's medical history in order to gauge your risks for certain hereditary diseases and conditions. At what age were these conditions diagnosed in a family member? Does anyone in your immediate family have recurrent headaches similar to yours? This is important because heredity can play a role in headache, particularly migraine.

Physical examination

Your doctor likely will examine your head, throat, eyes, ears and nose to check for signs and symptoms of illness or infection that may be causing your headache. He or she may also look for any neurological signs, such as vision problems or muscle weakness, that may indicate a secondary cause.

The medical history and physical examination are important elements of a diagnosis. They enable your doctor to select appropriate tests if he or she suspects a secondary cause for your headache. And they may indicate which medications and nonmedication strategies are appropriate for your treatment plan.

Initial diagnosis

Because the contributing factors to the different types of headaches are so complex and variable, coming up with an accurate diagnosis can be like piecing a puzzle together. Doctors may follow the classification system developed by the International Headache Society to help differentiate one headache type from another (see Chapter 2). The system provides specific details about each type of primary and secondary headache, including the frequency of attacks, the length of time each attack lasts, the characteristics of the head pain and the presence of accompanying signs and symptoms.

With such specific detail, it would seem that diagnosing a headache is a straightforward process for doctors — just check off the signs and symptoms until there's a match. And sometimes this is the case. Some headaches, such as cluster headache, have features that clearly set them apart from other types. But many headaches share signs and symptoms with only slight variation in the location of pain or in the frequency and duration of attacks, making them hard to diagnose. For example, diagnosis can be difficult when it comes to distinguishing between a tension-type headache and a mild migraine.

Some headaches may be the result of combined causes. Or it may be that you have more than one type of headache, and each type may require a separate diagnosis. For instance, some people experience a daily, mild to moderate headache (tension-type headache), as well as a more severe headache (migraine) that occurs several times a month.

In diagnosing the headache, your doctor will keep in mind any coexisting medical condition that could complicate your treatment. This information will have been related to your doctor in the medical history. For example, some people with migraine also have depression or anxiety, which can make headaches worse. It may be that your treatment plan will require you to resolve the emotional issues before your headaches can be managed effectively.

When additional testing is necessary

Sometimes, the cause of your headache remains uncertain or treatment seems to be ineffective. On these occasions, your doctor may recommend laboratory tests, such as a blood test or urine test, if he or she suspects a still undetermined medical condition is at the root of your problem.

For example, a blood test may confirm or rule out an infection that could be causing your headache. Your doctor also may want to check for certain thyroid or autoimmune conditions. Other serious disorders may need to be ruled out that, although rarely, can cause head pain.

Still, there's no laboratory test that can definitively diagnose a primary headache, for example, distinguishing a migraine from a tension-type headache. A clinical diagnosis is based primarily on your interview, medical history and physical examination.

Brain scans and other imaging tests

If you have an unusual or complicated headache, your doctor may order a brain scan to exclude serious causes of head pain that are sometimes difficult to detect, such as a brain tumor or hydrocephalus. Keep in mind, though, that very few headaches are actu-

Referral to a headache specialist

Frequently, the first physician to hear about your headache is a family doctor, and that's a good place to start. In many cases, your family doctor should be able to diagnose and treat a headache disorder.

On occasion, your headache pain may be difficult to categorize or treat. Your family doctor may feel your condition requires further expertise and may refer you to a specialist in treating headache. On the other hand, you may feel that your doctor isn't taking your condition seriously or is unable to meet your needs. On such occasions, you should feel free to consult a headache specialist yourself.

A headache specialist is most often a neurologist, a doctor who specializes in the brain and nervous system. Ideally, he or she will have extensive experience with headache care and will have dedicated a significant portion of his or her practice to treating people with headaches. Other doctors, such as some family physicians and internists, may also specialize in headache treatment.

So be aware that it may take more than one doctor to arrive at a correct diagnosis of your head pain, depending on your signs and symptoms and headache history. To find a neurologist near you, check with your local hospital or medical association, or you might try the yellow pages in your local telephone directory. If you contact a neurologist directly, be sure to ask if he or she specializes in headache management. The good news is that, with persistence, you and your doctor can begin taking steps to relieve a debilitating problem.

ally caused by conditions such as these. Imaging tests that doctors may use in the diagnosis of headache include:

X-rays. An X-ray is a simple procedure that uses radiation to make images of the internal structures of your body, including bones and organs. X-rays of your neck may reveal the development of arthritis or spinal problems that can contribute to headaches in rare instances.

Computerized tomography. Computerized tomography (sometimes called a CT or CAT scan) is an imaging procedure that uses a series of computer-directed X-rays. A CT scan of your head provides a cross-sectional view that helps doctors diagnose cranial tumors or infections. If there is concern about sinus disease, a CT scan of the sinuses can be revealing. A scan also can expose skull fractures, bleeding in the brain and other possible medical problems that may cause headache.

Magnetic resonance imaging. Magnetic resonance imaging (MRI) is a procedure that uses magnetism, radio waves and computer technology. A cranial MRI provides clear detailed information about the structure of your brain. MRI scans help doctors diagnose tumors, strokes, aneurysms, neurological diseases and other brain abnormalities. An MRI can also be used to examine the blood vessels that supply the brain.

Before a CT scan or MRI, you'll be asked to remove any objects on your body that contain metal, such as eyeglasses, jewelry or buckles, which might interfere with the procedure. You'll lie on a narrow table, with your head resting on a firm pillow. The table is positioned within an open, ring-shaped machine where the scanning takes place. You're asked to lie still during the procedure to keep the images clear.

Before either procedure, you may be given a special substance called a contrast agent, which is a dye. Typically, this agent is given intravenously, which means that it's injected into a vein in your arm. Contrast agents enhance the outlines of internal brain structures and certain types of abnormalities.

Other tests

Imaging tests can detect many, but not all, abnormalities that cause head pain. Depending on your signs and symptoms and headache history, your doctor may recommend one of these tests to further evaluate your headache:

Lumbar puncture. A lumbar puncture, also called a spinal tap, is often done when fever and stiff neck accompany a headache. It also may be used if your doctor is concerned about abnormally high or low pressure of your spinal fluid, bleeding around the brain, and infections such as meningitis or encephalitis. Any of these conditions can produce a headache. Because a lumbar puncture is an uncomfortable and invasive procedure, it's used only if your symptoms warrant it.

During the test, you may be asked to lie on your side, with your knees curled up toward your abdomen and your chin tucked to your chest. The skin covering your lower back is numbed with medication. A small, hollow needle is inserted into the skin and through a space between the vertebrae into the spinal canal, removing a sample of spinal fluid for testing in a laboratory. The procedure usually takes about 30 minutes. Headaches may be a complication of this procedure in some individuals, but the pain usually goes away after several hours or days.

Cerebral angiography. If your doctor suspects that the headache is caused by a blood vessel disorder, he or she may order a cerebral angiogram. This test produces an image of the blood vessels in your brain.

To start the procedure, the doctor injects a contrast agent into the arteries of your brain. Then, X-rays of your head are taken while you lie flat on an X-ray table. The X-rays, with the help of the dye, show blood flow through the targeted blood vessels and will reveal abnormalities in vessel walls. The entire procedure may take one to two hours to complete.

Why headache often goes undiagnosed

Despite important advances in the treatment of headache, many people needlessly tolerate severe or chronic head pain. Often, they endure the headache in silence. Why don't more people turn to their doctors for help?

For some people, fear prevents them from seeing a doctor. They assume that a debilitating headache occurs because something is seriously wrong and they don't wish to acknowledge the situation. Or they fear that the doctor will dismiss their headache as trivial. Other people mistakenly believe their headache is simply a fact of life and something to put up with. Some people never consult a doctor, preferring to treat the headache on their own — sometimes successfully, sometimes not.

Occasionally, a headache problem goes unrecognized, even when a person seeks medical care. Some doctors simply aren't familiar with headache disorders, so they may not be able to keep up with the advances in diagnosis and treatment. Or they just don't have the time in one office visit to thoroughly assess the problem. They may simply recommend self-care tips, such as reducing stress, and a prescription for pain medications without having identified the type of headache.

As noted, many factors can make headaches difficult to diagnose. For one, the manner in which a headaches develops is not always apparent, which can disguise the connections between certain symptoms. For another, secondary headaches have numerous possible causes — ranging from something as minor as caffeine withdrawal to something as serious as a brain tumor. In addition, many of the primary headaches have similar signs and symptoms. And some primary headaches can mimic secondary headaches or vice versa, further complicating matters.

Time to see your doctor?

Headache isn't something you should have to put up with, without the hope of relief. Anyone, including children, with severe, recurrent or unusual headaches should plan to consult a doctor. The good news is that, with professional assistance, your headache often can be effectively treated.

Getting an accurate diagnosis starts with your willingness to acknowledge the impact that a headache has on your life. Look for a doctor with whom you feel comfortable and who will work with you to find an effective treatment for pain. Some people who experience chronic headaches see more than one doctor before finding a specialist who can help them. But the rewards for their efforts can greatly enhance their quality of life.

Part 2

Migraine

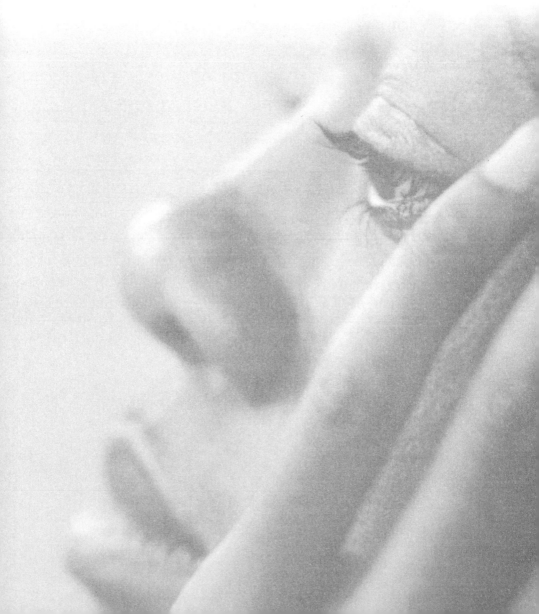

Chapter 4

Characteristics of migraine

Some people use the term *migraine* to describe just how intense their pain feels — a regular headache is just a headache, but a really bad headache is a migraine. To some extent, that's true. Migraines can be very painful. But migraine is actually a specific type of headache with well-defined characteristics that set it apart from other types of headaches. Among these characteristics are symptoms that often accompany the pain. These include nausea, vomiting, and sensitivity to light and sound. Often, the pain intensifies when you're physically active and is relieved by resting in a quiet, dark room.

Another important characteristic of migraine is its episodic nature — people with migraine (migraineurs) usually have many headaches over many years, but each attack is a distinct and separate event within the series. The frequency of the attacks varies from person to person. If you're an average migraineur, you probably experience one to two attacks a month.

According to the National Institutes of Health, migraine affects about 28 million Americans, 75 percent of whom are women. Usually people start having migraine between the ages of 10 and 46 years. Migraine has been studied far more than any other type of headache, which explains why much of the headache information you hear and read is about migraine.

Affliction of the ancients

By no means is migraine a modern illness. During the second century A.D. in Rome, the Greek physician Aretaeus wrote descriptions of a variety of diseases, including diabetes, epilepsy and migraine. To many who experience migraine today, this description will sound familiar:

There is much torpor, heaviness of head, anxiety, and weariness. For they flee the light; the darkness soothes their disease; nor can they bear readily to look upon or hear anything disagreeable.

The Greek physician Galen, a contemporary of Aretaeus, referred to the headache as *hemicranios*, or "half-head," describing the pain people often experienced on only one side of the head. As the word evolved, *hemicranios* transformed into the word *migraine* that we use today.

Types of migraine

According to the International Classification of Headache Disorders, to be diagnosed as having migraine, you will have had at least five headaches that meet the following criteria:

1. You've had attacks lasting from four to 72 hours.
2. Your head pain has at least two of these characteristics:
   - It's located on one side of your head.
   - It has a pulsating quality.
   - Its intensity is moderate to severe.
   - It's aggravated by routine physical activity.
3. At least one of these symptoms accompanies your headache:
   - Nausea or vomiting or both
   - Abnormal sensitivity to light and sound
4. Evaluations to find an underlying cause of your headache are normal, and no other disease can be considered a cause.

Headaches classified as migraine can be subdivided into several types, the most common of which are migraine with aura (formerly called classic migraine) and migraine without aura (formerly called common migraine). Other, less common variants exist.

Migraine with aura

About 30 percent of migraineurs experience what's known as an aura. Aura is a variety of sensations that come before, and sometimes accompany, the pain of a migraine attack. Like the word *migraine*, the word *aura* comes from the language of the ancient Greeks. It means "wind." And just as the wind often indicates an approaching storm, an aura signals an approaching migraine. The telltale characteristics of aura may include blind spots or bright flashes in your visual field, a numbing or tingling sensation in your skin, and muscular weakness. There may also be problems with the use or understanding of language (dysphasia).

Aura is closely associated with migraine. In other words, if you experience any of these phenomena before a headache, it's highly likely that you have a migraine. These criteria are used to diagnose migraine with aura:

1. You've had at least two headache attacks preceded by an aura.
2. The aura has at least three of the following characteristics:
   - Symptoms go away entirely between attacks.
   - Symptoms develop gradually over five minutes or more.
   - Symptoms last less than 60 minutes.
   - A headache starts within 60 minutes of the aura's disappearance, and in the interval between the aura and the headache you experience no symptoms. Less frequently, a headache begins during the aura.
3. Evaluations to find an underlying cause of your headache are normal, and no other disease can be considered a cause.

Aura sometimes disappears with age. It also may begin late in life, even if you've never had aura before a migraine in the past. For example, a female migraineur may start to experience aura after she begins to use oral contraceptives.

Migraine without aura

A migraine without aura isn't preceded by warning signs, although some people claim they can still feel a migraine attack coming on. For example, they may experience mood changes or a loss of appetite. Migraine without aura is more common than migraine with aura.

As noted, the nature of migraine attacks can change during a person's lifetime. Some people may start out with one type of migraine that evolves, over time, into another type. Other people may experience two types of migraine concurrently. Because of the shifting nature of these headaches, scientists debate whether migraine types are actually separate disorders or are different expressions of the same disorder.

Migraine variants

Other, rare forms of migraine exist, some accompanied by aura and others not. In fact, one type of migraine is characterized by aura with no head pain at all.

Basilar-type migraine. This is a migraine with aura that's thought to originate at the base of your brain (your brain stem). The aura may begin with visual disturbances in both your eyes, causing temporary blindness. This development may be followed by coordination problems, vertigo, ringing in your ears (tinnitus), double vision, nausea or vomiting, rapid, involuntary movement of your eyes (nystagmus), speech difficulties, tingling sensations on both sides of your body or loss of consciousness. Some studies show that basilar-type migraine is most common in young women. Attacks occur weeks or months apart and may be related to menstruation, stress or use of oral contraceptives. Over the years, the attacks tend to decrease.

Confusional migraine. This migraine with aura affects your brain's centers of consciousness in the cerebrum. People with confusional migraine are easily distracted and have difficulty with speech and motor skills. This state of general confusion may precede the headache or follow it, although the pain itself may be insignificant.

Retinal migraine. This type of migraine is a rare form of headache that includes aura. The visual disturbances and blind spots originate on your retina, the inner lining of your eye — unlike other forms of migraine with aura, in which the centers of your brain responsible for vision cause the disturbances. The aura of retinal migraine generally lasts several minutes and occurs in one eye rather than in both.

Hemiplegic migraine. The word *hemiplegia* refers to paralysis in one half of the body. Hemiplegic migraine involves the gradual onset of stroke-like symptoms with paralysis. It's usually accompanied by symptoms such as confusion, speech problems, tinnitus and vertigo. It can occur with or without aura. The symptoms may be part of the aura or they may follow the headache. The condition often begins in childhood and attacks may stop in adulthood.

Late-life migraine accompaniments. With this form of migraine, the visual disturbances of an aura occur, but there's no head pain. This condition often develops in older adults who have a history of migraine, but can happen even in older adults who have never had migraine before. A characteristic of late-life migraine is the presence of blind spots that slowly spread across your field of vision, although other sensory and motor difficulties may occur, as well as tingling or numbness. Late-life migraine accompaniments are not considered serious but seeing your doctor is advisable to eliminate the possibility of potentially serious problems.

Status migrainosus. This headache, which may or may not be accompanied by aura, is considered a rare complication rather than a type of migraine. Status migrainosus is a severely painful condition that lasts for more than 72 hours, sometimes for as long as a week. Usually the pain and nausea are so severe that hospitalization may be necessary. The headaches are especially dangerous if you become dehydrated from vomiting or diarrhea.

Ophthalmoplegic migraine. Although this condition was considered a migraine in the past, medical experts now believe that it's an inflammatory nerve condition. In the recent revision of the International Classification of Headache Disorders, it received a secondary headache designation (see Chapter 12).

Phases of a migraine

A migraine usually involves more than just the period of time when your head hurts. For adults, an attack may last anywhere from four to 72 hours. In fact, physicians have identified phases that unfold in sequence as the migraine develops. It's not necessary to experience all the phases in order for your headache to be a migraine, but most people experience more than one phase.

A typical migraine attack includes a premonitory phase, an aura phase, a headache phase and a postheadache phase. Some experts refine the sequence into more phases, and others simplify it into fewer phases.

Premonitory phase

Some migraineurs experience certain signs and symptoms — you might call them premonitions — that signal a migraine is coming on. These developments aren't the same thing as the aura, which tends to occur just before the headache begins and lasts only minutes. The premonitory phase, also called the prodrome, usually begins gradually and may last for several hours or for up to two days before the headache phase. Exactly how many migraineurs experience a premonitory phase is unknown, but it's believed that the phase is more common among migraineurs who experience aura and is more common among women than among men.

Premonitory signs and symptoms often go unnoticed. You could easily think you're just having a bad day. For example, the most common premonitory symptoms are feelings of depression, fatigue or weakness, difficulty with concentration, and a stiff neck. Anyone can experience these symptoms at one time or another and might not connect them to migraine attacks. Other symptoms may include frequent yawning, irritability, muscle ache, fluid retention and various gastrointestinal problems. In contrast, some migraineurs have increased energy and appetite (particularly for sweets), enhanced clarity of thought, and increased desire for work. Premonitory symptoms aren't always followed by a headache, or in some cases, a mild headache may develop that you don't consider a migraine.

Aura phase

Before the pain of a migraine starts, you may see stars or sparkling jagged patterns before your eyes, or you may have blind spots in your field of vision. This phenomenon, called a migraine aura, usually occurs in the 60 minutes preceding a migraine (see page C3 of the Color Section). It's not certain how many migraineurs experi-

Premonitory signs and symptoms

Some people regularly experience the same signs and symptoms before each migraine and can predict when the attack will happen. These premonitory signals may be psychological (affecting your emotions and moods), neurological (stemming from your nervous system), gastrointestinal (affecting your digestive system) or of a more general nature. Some of the more common signs and symptoms are listed below.

Psychological
- Depression
- Anxiety
- Irritability
- Hyperactivity
- Sluggishness
- Obsessive behavior

Gastrointestinal
- Hunger
- Food cravings
- Nausea
- Diarrhea
- Constipation
- Loss of appetite

Neurological
- Lack of concentration
- Yawning
- Trembling hands
- Sensitivity to light, sound or smell
- Blurred vision
- Dizziness

General
- Stiff neck
- Fatigue
- Thirst
- Goose bumps
- Shivering
- Achiness
- Increased urination

ence the aura phase. Some people have aura before every attack, whereas others experience only a few in their lifetimes. It appears to be more common in adults than in children.

Aura sensations may be mild or intense, and they may vary from attack to attack. Aura usually occurs about 20 minutes before the headache begins and generally lasts from 10 to 25 minutes before disappearing. Although aura will usually precede the headache, the two sometimes occur simultaneously. Still less commonly, aura may occur with no headache.

Visual disturbances are, by far, the most common feature of migraine aura. Descriptions of these disturbances vary:

- Stars, colorless dots, flashes of light, wavy lines or patterns that appear before your eyes and that often flicker or shimmer
- Blind spots that spread across your visual field
- Blurred, foggy vision
- Objects in your surroundings that appear as if they were shimmering in heat
- A crescent-shaped blind spot with a shimmering, white or gray, zigzagged border

Other types of aura symptoms may accompany the visual disturbances. There may be feelings of numbness or tingling in certain parts of your body. For example, a person often experiences tingling on one side of the mouth and in the same-side hand. These sensations may take 30 minutes to fully develop. Rarely, one-half of your body may become temporarily paralyzed for a few minutes. Speech difficulties and vertigo also may occur.

Occasionally, a person may experience abnormal perceptions of his or her surroundings — people and objects appear distorted or excessively large or small. These distortions of shape or size are sometimes termed an "Alice in Wonderland" syndrome because of the similarity to Lewis Carroll's fictional account in *Alice's Adventures in Wonderland.*

Between the end of the aura and the onset of head pain, there's usually a period of several minutes called a free interval. During this time, you may not have any visual disturbances, but you may feel lightheaded, sluggish or nauseated. You may also experience some anxiety and have difficulty speaking or thinking clearly.

Headache phase

The headache phase of migraine is characterized by throbbing or pounding head pain that's usually moderate to severe in intensity and aggravated by physical movement. In about 60 percent of attacks, the pain is on one side of the head (unilateral). In the remaining 40 percent of attacks, the pain is on both sides (bilateral).

Although migraine can start at any time of day, it frequently begins in the morning as a dull, steady ache that gradually builds

Aura before a migraine may start as a bright point of light in your visual field (middle) that develops into a shimmering, jagged crescent shape (bottom). The clouded area represents an expanding blind spot in your visual field.

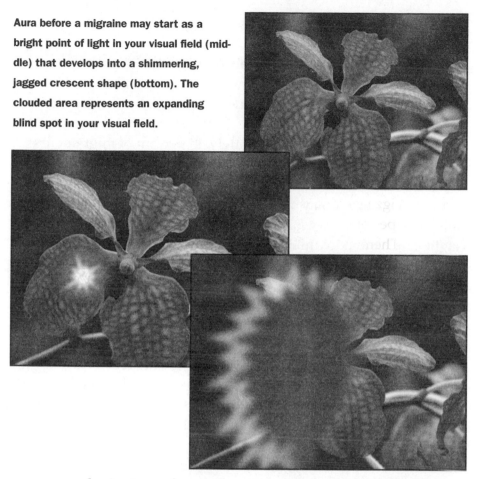

over several minutes or hours. In some people, the pain becomes disabling. For a majority of migraineurs, the headache lingers for less than a day.

You may find that pain intensity varies and that the pain may not always develop in the same location. The pain can switch from one side of the head to the other from attack to attack, or it may switch between unilateral and bilateral. Usually, the pain is focused on your forehead but any area of your head may be affected. Other signs and symptoms often accompany the head pain, including:

- **Nausea.** Almost 90 percent of all migraineurs are affected by nausea, and vomiting occurs in about one-third to one-half of adults with migraine.
- **Intolerance to light.** More that two thirds of migraineurs experience an extreme intolerance to light (photophobia),

which includes eye pain and an exaggerated sense of bright-
ness or glare.

- **Sensitivity to noise.** More than 70 percent of migraineurs
  experience unusual sensitivity to noise (phonophobia), such as
  conversation, traffic or even sounds such as nearby footsteps,
  causing discomfort and pain.
- **Aversion to odors.** Approximately 40 percent of migraineurs
  experience an aversion to certain smells, such as perfume,
  diesel exhaust or food aromas.

A migraine attack may also be accompanied by paleness of skin,
chills, profuse sweating, cold and clammy hands and feet, and
weight gain caused by fluid retention. Gastrointestinal problems,
such as diarrhea, constipation, bloating, belching or flatulence, may
develop. Other signs and symptoms include swelling or tenderness
of the scalp or face; bulging blood vessels in the temple; stiff neck;
difficulty concentrating and thinking clearly; feelings of depression,
fatigue, anxiety and irritability; and lightheadedness.

During the headache phase, many migraineurs retreat to a dark,
quiet room to be alone and rest. Since the pain tends to increase
with movement — even a slight tilt of the head — most people find
it best to lie or sit as still as possible until the pain subsides.

Although the headache phase generally is considered the pre-
dominant feature of a migraine, it's never the only feature. In fact,
some migraineurs may not even experience a headache phase.

Post-headache phase

How migraine ends will vary from one person to another and from
one attack to another. But all signs and symptoms of migraine disappear during the post-headache phase, permitting you to resume
normal routines. For many migraineurs, sleep signals the end of an
attack, whether a short nap or several hours of deep sleep. For others, the pain ends after vomiting. As the pain subsides, you may
feel disoriented, depressed, and emotionally and physically spent,
especially if you've experienced vomiting and diarrhea. There may
be scalp tenderness for a day or so after the attack. Some people
will feel listless and take a while to get back on their feet. Others
may feel unusually refreshed or elated.

Migraine triggers

Many people with migraine find that an attack will occur in response to a specific event or situation — for example, something they just ate, a particularly strong odor, a change in the weather or a stressful environment. These factors aren't necessarily the cause of migraine but they do seem to trigger the chain of events that results in a splitting headache.

It appears that a person with a genetic predisposition to migraine develops a sensitivity to something in the environment or within his or her own body that triggers the attack. Even though migraine may run in a family, different family members may have different triggers or no identifiable trigger at all. Furthermore, sensitivity to a certain factor may take years to develop.

To add to the complexity, the mere presence of a trigger isn't always enough to produce a migraine — rather, the trigger may be only one piece in a combination of genetic, biological, psychological and environmental factors at play. For example, eating chocolate may give you a migraine attack one day but not the next time you eat it because one of the other factors is missing.

Finding a migraine trigger takes time and effort, and you may never be able to identify any one trigger with certainty. But if you notice a correspondence between something you do and your headaches, you have identified a potential culprit. Avoiding that factor may help decrease the number of migraine attacks you have.

The list of reported migraine triggers is long. The most common ones include stress, diet, physical activity and hormonal changes.

Stress

Stress is one of the most commonly reported migraine triggers. A complex interaction between your biological and psychological makeup, stress may contribute to the onset of migraine attack or may prolong an existing headache.

There are two basic types of stress: major life events and daily hassles. Major life events include the death of a loved one, a change in career or a divorce. These are big events that require big adjustments. You're probably more than familiar with daily hassles, which range from searching for lost keys to dealing with traffic tie-ups to tolerating petty annoyances at work. Social commitments and finances may also contribute to daily stress.

Scientists believe that the small, everyday irritants may actually have a greater impact on headaches than big life events do. It's as if your body draws on unknown reserves of strength to deal with a crisis, whereas the routine, trifling events wear down your ability to cope. For some people, an inability to cope brings a headache.

Some people experience a migraine attack after the main period of stress has ended, such as after they've completed a project or while they're on vacation. This results in what is known as a let-down migraine. A variation of this headache is the weekend migraine, which may occur after a stressful work week. Other factors can contribute to weekend headaches, such as sleeping longer or drinking more alcohol.

Diet

Although many people report that certain foods trigger their migraine attacks, there are few scientific studies that prove a direct relationship. Migraine may require the interaction of several factors, with diet being just one of those factors. Here's a list of foods that are commonly reported as migraine triggers:

- Foods containing the naturally occurring chemical tyramine, such as aged cheese, dried herring, some sausages, sauerkraut, yeast extract, beers and ales on tap, and Chianti red wine
- Chocolate
- Citrus fruits
- Alcohol
- Overuse of caffeine-containing products
- The flavor enhancer monosodium glutamate (MSG) in certain brands of soy sauce, potato chips, salts and seasonings, and many fast foods
- Foods containing nitrate preservatives, including processed meats such as hot dogs, salami, pepperoni and sausages
- The artificial sweetener aspartame in certain brands of soda

Migraines can be the result of skipping meals, not eating enough, dieting or fasting. Scientists speculate that hunger combined with excessive activity or stress could trigger migraine. Missing the usual daily intake of caffeine also serves as a trigger.

Sleep

Migraine attacks are particularly common during normal sleep hours. One study found that as many as 48 percent of migraine attacks occurred between 4 a.m. and 9 a.m. Too much sleep or too little sleep can help trigger these attacks. This may contribute to the so-called weekend headache if your sleep routine changes over the weekends. Getting about the same amount of sleep every night of the week may help reduce the attacks.

Physical activity

Physical activity and exhaustion may trigger a migraine attack in people with a history of migraine. In most cases, the migraine is a result of activity that's more strenuous than usual or excessively prolonged. Other contributing factors may be exercising without warming up first, not drinking enough fluids, and exercising in locations that are at higher altitudes or higher temperatures than you're accustomed to.

Sexual activity can trigger a migraine in some people, especially men. The pain often begins abruptly during or before orgasm and may be accompanied by nausea and vomiting. Other types of headache, not necessarily migraine, can also result from sexual activity.

Hormonal changes

Hormonal changes in women have been linked to migraine. Around 60 percent of women who get migraine experience an attack right before, during or after a menstrual period, when hormone levels fluctuate.

For some women, the first migraine attack occurs during pregnancy. For other women, pregnancy tends to improve the condition, causing attacks to disappear completely or become milder or less frequent — especially in the last two trimesters. The use of oral contraceptives may likewise influence migraine attacks, either improving them or making them worse. Of course, there are women whose migraine seem unaffected by hormonal changes.

Changes in weather

Up to 78 percent of migraineurs say that weather changes can trigger migraine. Such changes include the passing of a cold front or warm front, thunderstorms, rising humidity, dry winds or a drop in atmospheric pressure (which can occur during a high-altitude flight or a trip to the mountains). Some people experience increased migraine attacks during certain seasons of the year.

Visual triggers

Intense sunlight and glare trigger headaches in about 30 percent to 45 percent of migraineurs. The reflection of the sun off snow, water or glass can be especially disturbing. Many migraineurs wear sunglasses to protect their eyes from this type of glare. Flickering lights, fluorescent bulbs, camera flashes and nighttime driving also are frequently reported migraine triggers.

Auditory triggers

Prolonged exposure to loud noise from traffic, construction equipment, machinery, tools and music concerts may trigger migraine. Even the noise of crowded shopping malls and large parties may cause a headache in some people.

Olfactory triggers

Various strong smells can be disturbing to migraineurs and cause headaches. Typically offensive odors include cigarette and cigar smoke, paint and exhaust fumes, detergents and chemical cleaners, newsprint, and colognes, perfumes and aftershaves. Personal toiletry fragrances can be overwhelming in a crowded elevator or on a commuter train. Public restrooms frequently have a strong detergent smell.

Motion sickness

Migraine appears to be linked to motion sickness, especially in children. Frequently, adult migraineurs have a history of motion sickness from childhood. People who have migraine with aura also seem to be more vulnerable to motion sickness. Many children have reported that their migraines occur whenever they travel.

Environmental factors

Environmental factors are occasionally identified as migraine triggers. These factors include air conditioning, office machinery, plastics, particleboard, vinyl and many other products.

Prescription medications

Certain prescription medications can cause migraine or aggravate an existing headache. Examples include:
- Heart and blood pressure medications, such as nitroglycerin
- Gastrointestinal medications, such as acid blockers
- Hormonal preparations, such as contraceptives and estrogens
- Certain antibiotics
- Certain nonsteroidal anti-inflammatory drugs

Talk to your doctor if you feel that any of your medications may be triggering migraine attacks. You may be able to find an alternative medication that won't cause your headaches.

Minor head trauma

Physical impacts or blows to the head, such as what may happen in sports, have been known to cause migraine. The headache usually occurs a few minutes after the trauma and is generally accompanied by nausea and vomiting. It may be preceded by aura.

Neck pain

Neck pain, for example from whiplash injuries, may cause migraine, even in someone who has never had one before. In fact, headache experts have found that certain locations in your neck and shoulder muscles, when subjected to pressure, can increase the pain of a current migraine.

Medical conditions

Various medical conditions have been associated with causing or aggravating migraine attacks. Migraineurs who also have chronic fatigue syndrome or fibromyalgia tend to have more frequent or more severe headaches. People with a history of migraine may experience migraine-type headaches when undergoing dialysis treatment for kidney problems.

A complicated relationship

Doctors are only beginning to unravel the intricacies of migraine. The interrelationships among various genetic, biological, psychological and environmental factors are complex. Yet even though an understanding of migraine remains incomplete, progress has been made in alleviating the severe symptoms of this type of headache. In the next few chapters, you'll find detailed information about migraine relief.

Chapter 5

Principles of medication therapy

Treatment of migraine can help reduce the frequency of your attacks, make the attacks less severe, prevent some attacks from happening and improve your ability to cope when attacks do occur. For the most effective outcome, the treatment should be a team effort between you and your doctor. And this team effort should begin with a proper diagnosis and an accurate history of your headache.

The headache history collects information about the symptoms you're experiencing and about the way pain is affecting your life. The information may be gathered during the initial doctor visit in a written questionnaire or directly during a one-on-one interview. The history helps the doctor make a diagnosis and serves as a base line for later assessments of your condition (for more information on the headache history, see Chapter 3).

The doctor will base much of your treatment on how frequent or severe your signs and symptoms are and which are the most both-ersome. It's also important for your doctor to know from the diag-nosis whether another medical condition is causing your head-ache. Taking migraine medications when your headache is caused by something else, such as infection, can be dangerous. Pain relief may disguise the true reason for the pain and prevent proper treat-ment for a serious, perhaps even life-threatening, problem.

When it comes to migraine treatment, one size does not fit all. There are many effective options — it's just that certain options work well for some migraineurs and not for others. Sometimes you and your doctor may have to try more than one type of medication or lifestyle change before deciding on the right treatment or the right combination of treatments. But with time and patience, successful management of migraine attacks can usually be achieved.

Types of treatment

Treatment of migraine involves two major strategies: lifestyle management and drug therapy. You'll read about lifestyle management — which includes maintaining regular sleep patterns, eating a healthy diet, getting enough exercise, avoiding stress and making modifications to some of your behaviors — later in Chapter 7. This chapter introduces the principles of drug therapy, which is often the starting point in a migraine treatment plan. The details on specific migraine medications are provided in Chapter 6.

When using drug therapy, it's important to know what a medication is intended to do and what improvements you may expect from taking it. If you expect it to cure your migraine completely, you're bound for disappointment. But there are plenty of medication choices available that, when combined with lifestyle management, can keep migraine under control and prevent attacks from interfering too much with your daily life. Doctors generally classify headache treatment in two ways: acute and preventive.

Acute treatment

The goal of acute treatment is rapid relief. It's usually taken to diminish or stop the pain of a migraine attack once the headache has started. Acute treatment generally involves medication, often in the form of general pain relievers or medications targeted specifically at migraine. Certain lifestyle measures may also help achieve short-term relief (see Chapter 7), but they're usually more helpful for headache prevention. If you have nausea and vomiting, you may also take acute medications to relieve those symptoms.

In the past, doctors often started migraineurs with the safest, least expensive drugs and then progressed to more aggressive treatments if the initial ones didn't work. Today, many doctors prefer a customized approach — beginning treatment with what's considered to be most effective, based on the severity of an individual's signs and symptoms. For example, if your attacks are disabling, your doctor may start with a prescription for a strong, highly effective medication. If your headache is mild or moderate, over-the-counter pain relievers may be sufficient to ease the pain.

If a drug provides only partial relief for your headache, your doctor may consider adding another drug to take along with the first medication. This combination of drugs may improve the effectiveness of your treatment. If nausea is a problem, your doctor may also recommend taking an anti-nausea agent (antiemetic) to help keep oral medications in your system.

Your doctor may also prescribe a backup or rescue medication for especially painful attacks, when your regular medications aren't able to provide relief. If nausea or vomiting prevents you from taking medications orally, your doctor may prescribe a nasal spray, injection or suppository form of pain relief.

In order to get the most out of your acute medications, it's important that you follow these basic principles:

Start acute treatment early in a migraine attack. You want to cut your headache "off at the pass," so to speak, before it gets too painful. If you have an aura before your headache, you may wish to begin treatment then. Most oral medications are less effective after an attack has started because your body is not able to absorb the drugs quickly, and fully developed pain is harder to turn off. But keep in mind that a sumatriptan injection isn't effective until after a headache begins.

Take your medication in the correct dosage and formulation. It's important to take the correct dosage of any drug, whether it's prescription or over-the-counter. If your current dosage is not providing relief, talk to your doctor about safely increasing the dose or finding another medication. Before you leave your doctor's office, make sure you understand when to take each medication and how much medication to take. If you frequently experience vomiting

Rebound headaches

You feel a headache coming on, so you reach for an over-the-counter pain reliever or a medication that your doctor has prescribed. That's what you're supposed to do, right? Right, but if you find yourself taking pain medication more than two or three days a week, you're likely contributing to your headaches rather than easing them.

Overuse of headache medications — using more than the label instructs or your doctor prescribes — produces its own kind of headache. Doctors call it medication-induced headache or, more commonly, rebound headache. As your body becomes accustomed to the effects of a medication that's taken frequently, any slight change may cause your headache to return, or rebound, sometimes more intensely than before. Overuse of medication may also lower the point at which you experience pain — your pain threshold.

Rebound headaches tend to occur daily, beginning shortly after your medication has worn off. They may even be continuous throughout the day, though these usually aren't severe. Signs and symptoms that may accompany rebound headaches include nausea, anxiety, restlessness, irritability, memory problems, difficulty concentrating and depression.

Breaking the rebound cycle requires you to reduce or stop taking pain medication — which can be difficult to do on your own. Start by alerting your doctor that you have a problem. Some people are embarrassed to do so because they feel the problem is similar to dependence on an illegal drug. This isn't the case — the drug is legal and the dependence is a result of frequent headaches.

When you stop taking the medication, you may go through a period of increased headaches before things get better. Sometimes, if the headaches are severe, hospitalization may be necessary. After you've broken the cycle, you and your doctor can find a safer way to manage your condition. One method may be long-term preventive therapy, which will help control migraine attacks without contributing to rebound headaches.

during a migraine attack, your doctor may prescribe a nonoral drug, such as a nasal spray, suppository or injection, which allows the medication to stay in your system.

Give your treatment a chance. Generally, two or three migraine attacks need to be treated with a certain drug or drug dose before you're able to assess whether the treatment is effective or not.

Limit use of acute medications to two or three days a week. If your body becomes accustomed to the effect of a certain drug, withdrawal from the drug — even for a few hours — can result in a headache. When a rebound headache develops, your first reaction is to take more pain medication (see sidebar "Rebound headache"). The result is a hurtful cycle that isn't easy to break. If you have very frequent migraine attacks, preventive therapy may help you avoid the overuse of acute medications.

Preventive treatment

Preventive measures are taken to stop headaches from happening. They also may reduce the duration of an attack or diminish the intensity of pain when a migraine occurs. Whereas acute treatment is effective when taken at the time of an attack, preventive treatment is taken at intervals, whether or not you have a headache. Preventive strategies frequently combine medications and lifestyle management. It's rare that preventive efforts eliminate headaches completely, but they can make your condition less disabling and improve your responsiveness to acute treatment.

Migraine medication can be used in different ways for short-term prevention. You may take medication whenever your body gives you clear warning signs that an attack is near, for example during the premonitory phase of a migraine attack. Or you can be preemptive, for example, taking medication a few hours before you're exposed to circumstances that you know will trigger a migraine, such as before you participate in intense exercise.

Medication can also be used when you know you'll be going through a limited time of increased risk. For instance, you may take preventive medications for a few days before you get your period if you have menstruation-related headaches or before you travel to a high-altitude area if changes in air pressure cause your headaches.

Long-term prevention differs from the short-term approach because it involves taking medication over several months or even years. The drug is usually taken on a daily basis. You may consider long-term prevention if:

- Acute medication doesn't provide sufficient relief or doesn't work at all.
- Your migraine attacks are frequent and you risk overusing acute medications.
- Overuse of acute medications leads to rebound headaches.
- Migraine seriously disrupts your ability to function.
- The side effects of acute treatment are bothersome, even if the treatment effectively stops pain.
- Migraine carries serious risks such as stroke, which may cause permanent injury to your nervous system.
- You prefer to have as few migraine attacks as possible.

If you're on some form of preventive therapy, you can still use acute medications when a migraine attack occurs. Avoid preventive therapy during pregnancy, as the medications may have an effect on your unborn baby — unless your signs and symptoms are so severe that the benefits of medication outweigh the risks. This is an issue to discuss with your doctor.

Although there are many preventive medications available, you and your doctor will determine which course of ongoing treatment is best suited for you. Most drug prescriptions for preventing migraine follow a similar pattern:

- Medication starts at a low dose in order to reduce the likelihood of side effects.
- If needed, the dose may be increased gradually to be more effective.
- Treatment may continue at a dose that's considered safe and effective for up to three months. At that point, the quality of treatment is assessed and a decision will be made to either maintain or change the dose.
- All use of medications that could interfere with migraine treatment are avoided. If overuse of an acute medication produces rebound headaches, for example, preventive drugs will not work until that medication is no longer taken.

Headache diary

A useful tool that doctors often recommend to migraineurs is a headache diary. A headache diary is a type of journal in which you describe each headache attack, as well as the circumstances surrounding the attack. You may include entries only for those days that you have a headache, recording information from at least three attacks, preferably in succession.

One goal of a headache diary is to help you understand the nature of your migraines attacks over time. Your diary may answer questions such as: How frequently does your headache occur in a month? Does it always start in the same way? What time of day does it generally occur? Is the pain always the same, or does it vary from one attack to another? What types of actions or situations seem to make them worse?

Perhaps an even more important goal, the diary can help you and your doctor evaluate the effectiveness of your headache treatment. Is there a noticeable change in your headache since you started taking medications or developing better sleep habits? Does treatment make it easier to cope with your headache and function in everyday activities? Does treatment work effectively every time you use it? Are there any side effects of medication? How bothersome are those side effects?

Headache diaries are available in different styles and formats. Nevertheless, most diaries register the following information:

- When and how the headache attack began
- How long the attack lasted
- Where the pain was located and how severe it was
- What type of treatment you used and how well it worked

Keeping a headache diary that registers this type of information compliments the details in your headache history. This, in turn, allows your treatment to be further customized to your needs. That's why it's so important to keep the diary, especially after you've started treatment. If your treatment isn't satisfactory, you and your doctor can look for ways to improve it.

Many people closely monitor their headache diaries to help them identify potential migraine triggers. This is certainly a worthwhile exercise because avoiding known triggers can help decrease the frequency of migraine attacks. At the same time, triggers can be hard to identify. Too many migraineurs end up on severely restricted diets in an effort to avoid any and all potential triggers, including those that may not even affect them.

Following up on your treatment plan

Treatment for migraine often requires a bit of refining before the best approach is established. So don't give up if you don't succeed on the first try. You'll likely need a follow-up appointment with your doctor to assess the effectiveness of your treatment.

Bring your headache diary with you to the follow-up appointment. It provides a basis for discussion with your doctor and reminds you of things you may otherwise forget to mention. Discuss any changes you wish to make to your treatment plan with your doctor before you attempt to make them. Some medications take a while before they have an impact, and you just may need to carry on with them for a little longer. Remember, the teamwork between you and your doctor is one of the best ways to manage migraine.

Chapter 6

Medications

In Chapter 5 you learned about the general principles of medication therapy. This chapter deals with specific acute and preventive drugs, including the different classes of medications that are available and possible side effects that each medication may have. Chapter 7 will discuss many of the nondrug therapies that people use to supplement a treatment program.

In the past, aspirin was often the recommended choice of headache medication. Today aspirin remains a treatment option, but other headache drugs have been developed, some of them specifically designed for migraine. In addition, drugs that generally are used to treat other conditions, such as high blood pressure or depression, have been found useful in treating headaches. In short, a much wider selection of migraine medications is available today.

It's important to understand the role of medications in your treatment program and their relationship to other strategies you may be using. They must be taken at prescribed times and at appropriate strengths and dosages to get the best results.

In addition, it's essential to work with your doctor to get an accurate diagnosis of your headache so that your treatment can be targeted at the correct problem. Remember that the goals of treatment are effective short-term relief and long-term management of your headache.

Acute pain relief

Acute treatment tries to alleviate migraine symptoms as early in the attack as possible. The treatment is aimed at relieving not only head pain but also symptoms such as nausea and vomiting. Several classes of drugs are used for acute treatment, ranging from general pain relievers to medications specific to migraine (See the list of acute medications on page 63). The choice of medication will depend on how severe and frequent your headaches are, what your associated signs and symptoms are, whether you have any other medical conditions, and what has or hasn't worked for you in the past. Your doctor can help you make the best choice.

Analgesics

Analgesics, or pain relievers, are often the first line of treatment for headache. Because most analgesics are available over the counter and are easy to buy, they're some of the most widely used headache medications. For people with mild to moderate migraine pain, these drugs may provide sufficient relief.

Analgesics should be taken as early in the attack as possible to be most effective. You may have discovered that taking an analgesic along with caffeine can be helpful, such as taking aspirin with a cup of coffee. A few drugs contain caffeine already (Excedrin).

If analgesics aren't giving you adequate relief, discuss other options with your doctor. More than half the people with disabling headaches use only over-the-counter drugs, although they might benefit more from prescription drugs. One reason some people avoid seeing the doctor is so they don't have to admit to themselves that the condition is serious. But if headaches are interrupting your ability to function in daily life, it's important to take the best possible care of this condition. A prescription drug may provide more relief than you thought possible.

Side effects and cautions. Analgesics are usually well tolerated, and their side effects are relatively few. But taking them more than two or three days a week can lead to medication overuse. Extended use of nonsteroidal anti-inflammatory drugs (NSAIDs), including aspirin, can cause upset stomach, nausea, vomiting, and gastric irri-

---

Dealing with nausea and vomiting

If you experience nausea or vomiting with your migraine attacks, talk to your doctor about taking an anti-nausea agent or antiemetic (an-tee-uh-MET-ik), along with your headache medication. Chlorpromazine (Thorazine), hydroxyzine (Vistaril), metoclopramide (Octamide, Reglan, others) and promethazine (Phenergan) are examples of antiemetics. These drugs can alleviate nausea symptoms but may make you feel drowsy. If you're having difficulty taking oral medications because of nausea or vomiting, your doctor may prescribe a drug in the form of a nasal spray, injection or suppository, which can help keep the drug in your system.

---

tation and bleeding. If you have a history of ulcers, gastritis or kidney disease, you may not be able to take NSAIDs at all.

Because aspirin can interfere with your blood's clotting ability, avoid using it if you have a bleeding disorder or if you're taking blood-thinning medications. Acetaminophen doesn't cause the same gastric or bleeding side effects as aspirin, and so it may be a suitable alternative to aspirin and other NSAIDs.

If you're pregnant, avoid the use of aspirin, particularly in the last three months of pregnancy, as it may cause problems with the heart or blood flow of the fetus. Overuse of aspirin can cause low birth weight and even death of the baby.

Triptans

Triptans are a major advance in migraine treatment. For many people with severe migraine attacks, triptans are the drug of choice (see page C8 of the Color Section). Triptans are effective in relieving the pain, nausea and sensitivity to light and sound that are associated with this headache. Overall, they're well-tolerated medications with few side effects. However, these drugs are not recommended for basilar-type migraine or hemiplegic migraine.

Since the introduction of sumatriptan in the 1990s — the initial product in this drug class — a series of related medications have become available. All of these drugs are produced as oral tablets.

Sumatriptan and zolmitriptan are available as nasal sprays, and sumatriptan also in injection form. Relief occurs within two hours in about 60 percent of people who use tablets, which usually are prescribed if migraine onset is gradual. The spray and injectable forms deliver more of the drug to the bloodstream in less time and are most often used when rapid pain relief is necessary. Symptom relief occurs nearly 80 percent of the time with injections.

Unlike most migraine medications, which are taken as early in the attack as possible, triptans are administered after head pain begins. The injectable sumatriptan hasn't proved as effective when taken during the aura phase. Lying down in a quiet, dark room after you take the medication may help relieve pain.

Side effects and cautions. Side effects of triptans include nausea, chest pressure, drowsiness, dizziness and fatigue, but most of these symptoms go away in less than an hour. In rare cases, people taking sumatriptan have developed an allergic reaction that requires medical attention. The injectable form of sumatriptan may cause irritation at the injection site. To help your doctor determine what's causing any side effects, be sure he or she knows all of the medications you're taking.

Recurring headaches can also be a problem for some people who treat an initial headache with triptans. The recurring headaches usually develop within several hours of administering the first dose of medication. But recurrences are less frequent when the headaches are treated early, and those headaches that do develop usually respond well to a second dose of a triptan or to a dose of analgesics. Rebound headaches also may occur. As a general rule, to avoid rebound headaches, don't use triptans regularly for more than two days a week.

Other possible side effects of triptans, although rare, include stroke and heart attack. Therefore, people with conditions such as uncontrolled high blood pressure and coronary artery disease or a history of heart attack should not take these drugs. If you have any risk factors for coronary artery disease, including being over the age of 40, your doctor may recommend that you undergo heart tests to confirm that no disease is present. In addition, triptans have not yet been proved safe during pregnancy.

Acute medications for migraine

Analgesics

Acetaminophen (Tylenol, others)

Acetaminophen, aspirin and
caffeine (Excedrin)

Nonsteroidal anti-inflammatory
drugs (NSAIDs)

- Aspirin
- Diclofenac potassium
  (Cataflam)
- Ibuprofen (Advil, Motrin)
- Indomethacin (Indocin)
- Ketorolac tromethamine
  (Toradol)
- Naproxen (Aleve,
  Naprosyn, others)
- Piroxicam (Feldene)

COX-2 inhibitors

- Celecoxib (Celebrex)
- Rofecoxib (Vioxx)
- Valdecoxib (Bextra)

Triptans

Almotriptan (Axert)

Eletriptan (Relpax)

Frovatriptan (Frova)

Naratriptan (Amerge)

Rizatriptan (Maxalt)

Sumatriptan (Imitrex)

Zolmitriptan (Zomig)

Ergots

Dihydroergotamine (D.H.E. 45,
Migranal)

Ergotamine (Ergomar)

Ergotamine and caffeine (Cafergot,
Wigraine)

Butalbital combinations

Butalbital and acetaminophen
(Phrenilin)

Butalbital, acetaminophen and caffeine (Fioricet, Esgic, others)

Butalbital, aspirin and caffeine
(Fiorinal)

Opiate combinations

Codeine and acetaminophen
(Tylenol #3, Tylenol #4)

Hydrocodone and acetaminophen
(Vicodin, Vicodin ES)

Oxycodone and acetaminophen
(Percocet, Tylox)

Oxycodone and aspirin (Percodan)

Propoxyphene and acetaminophen
(Darvocet-N 100, Darvon
Compound 65)

Corticosteroids

Dexamethasone (Decadron)

Methylprednisolone (Medrol)

Prednisone (Deltasone, Sterapred)

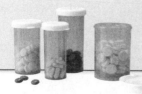

Ergots

Ergotamine has been around for nearly 70 years, and it was a common prescription choice for migraine before triptans were introduced. It's available as an oral tablet, but it also comes in a suppository form.

An advantage of ergotamine is that it's fairly inexpensive compared with triptans. But several limitations restrict its use and make it less effective than triptans. For one thing, the drug is poorly absorbed in your system, especially when you take it orally. For another, you must take it as soon as the pain starts in order for it to work well. In addition, appropriate dosages vary greatly from person to person, leading to a trial-and-error approach until the right dosage is found.

Dihydroergotamine is an ergot derivative that may be a better alternative to ergotamine for many people. It has fewer side effects and can be administered through a nasal spray or an injection — it's not effective when taken orally. Studies indicate that dihydroergotamine is consistently more effective than ergotamine, and is associated with a low risk of headache recurrence.

Side effects and cautions. Nausea and vomiting are common side effects of ergotamine, but less common with dihydroergotamine. Your doctor may prescribe an antiemetic for you to help control the nausea. Other side effects include dizziness, tingling or prickling sensations, abdominal cramps, chest tightness, flushing, restlessness and anxiety.

Overuse of either medication can lead to rebound headaches, especially with ergotamine. As a result, both drugs are used primarily for infrequent headaches that don't respond to triptans.

As with the triptans, these medications aren't recommended for people who have coronary artery disease or any condition that affects your blood vessels. If you have any cardiac risk factors, your doctor may recommend that you undergo cardiac testing before taking an ergot.

People who should not use ergots include pregnant women and women who are breast feeding their children, as well as individuals with malnutrition, hyperthyroidism, infection and fever. Avoid ergots if you've used triptans within the previous 24 hours.

Butalbital combinations

Medications that combine the sedative butalbital with aspirin or acetaminophen are sometimes used to treat migraine attacks. Some combinations also include caffeine or codeine. In general, no one should use butalbital combinations more than one day a week because of the high risk of rebound headaches and withdrawal symptoms. They're generally recommended when a less problematic drug can't be used or isn't effective.

Side effects and cautions. Common side effects include drowsiness, fatigue, nausea and lightheadedness. Feelings of euphoria or high spirits also are common. Butalbital combinations can impair your motor skills, so don't take them if you'll be driving or operating heavy machinery within the following hours.

People recovering from alcohol or drug abuse, or who have a history of medication overuse, should avoid butalbital combinations because of the risk of addiction. Those who have depression also should not use these drugs.

Opiates and opiate combinations

Opiates — narcotics — are another drug class that may be used to treat migraine pain. They're potent pain relievers and may be prescribed when people can't take triptans or ergots because of a medical condition or because of side effects. They're often a last-resort option and used only for short term or for infrequent attacks. Opiates may serve as backup medication when an attack is severe.

Codeine is a commonly used opiate and often taken in addition to a simple analgesic, such as aspirin or acetaminophen. More potent opiates, such as propoxyphene or hydrocodone, may be used alone or in combination with simple analgesics.

Side effects and cautions. Constipation is the most common side effect of opiates. Other side effects include euphoria (or the opposite — unhappiness), drowsiness, confusion, dizziness, nausea, vomiting and itchiness. A low dose of an antihistamine such as diphenhydramine (Benadryl) may help to relieve the itchiness.

To reduce the serious risk of medication overuse, opiates should be limited to no more than one or two days a week. People with a history of drug or alcohol problems should avoid using opiates.

Corticosteroids

This class of drugs is commonly used to treat asthma, rheumatoid arthritis and other inflammatory conditions. Although scientists aren't sure why or how it occurs, short courses of drugs such as methylprednisolone, prednisone and dexamethasone have been known to relieve headache pain. Because corticosteroids take time to act, they're most often used for prolonged migraine or as emergency treatment for status migrainosus — a migraine that lasts for 72 hours or more.

Side effects and cautions. Prolonged use of corticosteroids can lead to serious side effects, including an increased risk of osteoporosis. Corticosteriods are used with caution in people with diabetes because these drugs can increase blood sugar levels. For these reasons, corticosteroids are used only for short periods of time and usually only when other methods have failed.

Preventive therapy

Migraine prevention helps control headaches before they happen. You take preventive medications at regular intervals, not just when you have a headache, to reduce the frequency, severity, and duration of migraine attacks. Preventive strategies can be used on a short-term or long-term basis. Sometimes, they're pre-emptive in nature, taken only when you know an attack is imminent.

Preventive therapy may be an option if you have two or more debilitating headaches a month or a need to use pain-relieving medications more than twice a week. Prevention is also important when acute pain medications aren't helping or when you have an uncommon form of migraine that puts you at risk of further complications, such as hemiplegic migraine.

Various types of medications have been found to be helpful for preventing migraine and other types of headache, although most of these drugs were developed to treat other health conditions. Taking medications to prevent migraine is different from taking medications to relieve a migraine attack. For one thing, preventive medications usually are taken on a daily basis instead of a need-only basis.

For another thing, the benefits of preventive drugs aren't always immediately obvious. Generally, it takes awhile — sometimes up to three months — before the benefits are noticeable.

For preventive therapy to be effective, you should take medication exactly as prescribed even when you feel you may not need it. Keep in mind that overuse of acute pain medication can interfere with the effectiveness of preventive drugs. Preventive therapy generally isn't recommended for pregnant women. Before prescribing preventive medications, your doctor may wish to verify that you're on adequate birth control if you're a woman of childbearing age.

Beta blockers

Beta blockers were developed to treat coronary artery disease and were approved later for treatment of high blood pressure. Studies now indicate that a number of beta blockers are effective in the prevention of migraine, although researchers aren't sure why.

Side effects and cautions. Common side effects of beta blockers are fatigue and a reduced capacity for strenuous physical activity. Other side effects may include cold hands, sleep problems, loss of sex drive, impotence, memory disturbance and depression.

Beta blockers aren't recommended for people who have asthma and chronic obstructive pulmonary disease because the beta blockers may interfere with certain factors important to breathing. Other health disorders that may limit the use of beta blockers include congestive heart failure, Raynaud's disease, type 1 diabetes (formerly called insulin-dependent diabetes), slow heart rate (bradycardia) and low blood pressure.

Anti-seizure medications

Clinical studies have found that a number of anti-seizure drugs (anticonvulsants) can effectively prevent migraine. In fact, divalproex (Depakote) is one of the few preventive drugs for migraine that has no cardiovascular effects and thus is especially well suited for people who can't take beta blockers. It's also a drug of choice for athletes with migraines because it doesn't affect their ability to exercise. Other anti-seizure drugs used for migraine prevention include gabapentin and topiramate.

Side effects and cautions. High doses of divalproex can lead to nausea, vomiting, diarrhea, drowsiness and weakness. Other side effects may include weight gain, hair loss, tremor and indigestion. The drug isn't recommended for headaches in children under 10 years of age (although it may be used for seizures in children) or anyone who has a history of liver disease. Divalproex can also cause birth defects, so it's not safe to use during pregnancy.

Side effects of topiramate and gabapentin include dizziness, drowsiness, fatigue, and difficulty concentrating. Topiramate may cause weight loss and prickling or tingling sensations. Kidney stones develop in a small percentage of people taking topiramate, so it's important to drink plenty of fluids to minimize this risk.

Antidepressants

Certain antidepressants are helpful in preventing headaches such as migraine. Most effective are the tricyclic antidepressants, especially if you have frequent migraine or a mixture of migraine and tension-type headache. You don't have to have depression to take these drugs for migraine prevention, but they can serve a dual purpose if you have both conditions.

Certain other antidepressants, such as the selective serotonin reuptake inhibitor (SSRI) fluoxetine (Prozac), have proved mildly useful in treating migraine in people who also have depression or anxiety. Monoamine oxidase inhibitors (MAOIs) also have been used for a similar purpose, but MAOI use is limited because of serious side effects and the complex management required.

Side effects and cautions. The side effects of tricyclic antidepressants are generally mild to moderate, including sleepiness, dry mouth, constipation, urinary retention, blurred vision, increased appetite with weight gain and excessive sweating. Another fairly common side effect is postural hypotension — a feeling of faintness caused by a sudden drop in blood pressure when you stand up too quickly. Tremor and agitation are less common. Sexual dysfunction can occur with SSRIs, but may be treated with other drugs.

Tricyclic antidepressants aren't recommended for people with uncontrolled seizures. They can increase your heart rate, which limits their use in people with certain cardiovascular disorders.

> **Preventive medications for migraine**
> Drugs to prevent migraine are taken at regular intervals, often daily, whether you have a headache or not.
>
> **Beta blockers**
> Atenolol (Tenormin)
> Metoprolol (Lopressor, Toprol)
> Nadolol (Corgard)
> Propranolol (Inderal)
> Timolol (Blocadren)
>
> **Calcium channel blockers**
> Verapamil (Calan, Covera, Isoptin)
>
> **Anti-seizure drugs**
> Divalproex (Depakote)
> Gabapentin (Neurontin)
> Topiramate (Topamax)
>
> **Antidepressants**
> Amitriptyline (Elavil)
> Nortriptyline (Aventyl, Pamelor)
> Protriptyline (Vivactil)

Calcium channel blockers

These cardiovascular drugs are commonly used to lower blood pressure but have also been useful in preventing migraine, particularly in people who can't take beta blockers because of a condition such as asthma or Raynaud's disease. Verapamil is perhaps the most widely used calcium channel blocker for migraine prevention.

Side effects and cautions. A common side effect of verapamil is constipation, but the drug may also cause dizziness and flushing. In addition, verapamil slows your heart rate, so it's not recommended if you have congestive heart failure, heart block, irregular heartbeat or bradycardia, or if you're already using beta blockers.

Anti-serotonin agents

Certain drugs that block the effects of the brain chemical serotonin have proved useful in preventing migraine. Methysergide (Sansert) had a good success rate in preventing migraine but is no longer available in the United States. Cyproheptadine is generally used to prevent migraine in children. Common side effects of cyproheptadine include drowsiness, dizziness, blurred vision, dry mouth, increased appetite and weight gain.

On the horizon

Although a variety of migraine medications are available, many have limitations to their use — either because other medical conditions prevent it or because the side effects can't be tolerated. Headache researchers continue to look for the ideal medication that would be almost universally effective and has few side effects.

Botulinum toxin

You may recognize botulinum toxin type A by its brand name Botox — the popular, wrinkle-smoothing wonder drug. In recent years, people who received Botox treatment for forehead wrinkles also noted improvement of their headaches. Researchers picked up on this anecdotal evidence and undertook studies to test the effects of botulinum toxin type A on different types of headaches.

Preliminary data indicate that botulinum toxin may indeed provide acute pain relief and long-term headache prevention. The effects of a single treatment of botulinum toxin on headaches can last for about three months. In addition, the drug doesn't appear to have many of the side effects commonly experienced with other headache medications.

Currently, there's not enough evidence to recommend use as a first-line therapy for migraine. But until additional studies are completed, it may be an appropriate alternative for people who haven't had success with other migraine medications.

Take an active role

To get the most from your medications, it's important to take an active role in your headache care. This means helping to create a medication plan, sharing information openly, watching for problems and asking for help when you need it. Whether it's OTC or prescription drugs you're taking, learn both their brand names and generic names, and understand how each drug fits into your plan. And make sure you know the correct dosage, formulation and schedule for each medication.

Anatomy of the brain

Meninges

Protecting the central nervous system are three layers of membrane called the meninges. The tough outer layer is called the dura mater and the delicate inner layer is the pia mater. The middle layer is the arachnoid, a weblike structure filled with fluid that cushions the brain.

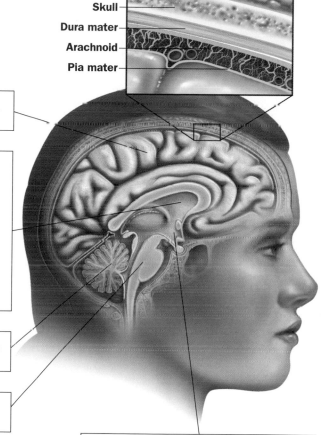

Skull
Dura mater
Arachnoid
Pia mater

Cerebral cortex

Thalamus

The thalamus interprets incoming pain messages and relays the messages to specialized regions of the brain, primarily in the cerebral cortex.

Cerebellum

Brainstem

Hypothalamus

Below the thalamus is the hypothalamus, a region of the brain that helps regulate many vital body processes and may be involved in the onset of cluster headache.

Migraine

Scientists are uncertain about all the factors involved in a migraine attack but this figure illustrates one interpretation of the process. A migraine is thought to occur when the brain's neural pathways for pain are activated abnormally — meaning pain messages are registered in the brain despite the fact that there's no external source for the pain.

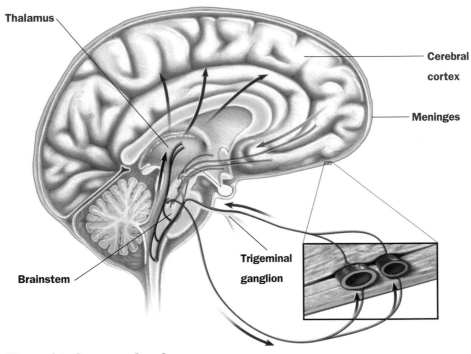

How migraine may develop

- Pain messages travel along neural pathways (red arrow) leading from the meninges, the outer covering of the brain, to the trigeminal ganglion. From there, the messages follow the main pathway of the trigeminal nerve into the brainstem and circulate among different nuclei there.
- From the brainstem, many of the messages are sent to the thalamus (purple arrow), which, in turn, relays information to locations in the cerebral cortex. At this point in the process, headache pain registers in your consciousness. The various cortical locations communicate back to the brainstem (green arrow).
- The brainstem nuclei attempt to modulate or diminish the incoming pain messages in a reflex action. Neural signals travel back along different pathways to blood vessels in the meninges (blue arrow), causing the vessels to dilate. As the pain messages diminish, head pain disappears.

Migraine aura

Visual disturbances are the most common symptoms of aura, the migraine phase that may occur prior to the onset of head pain. The disturbances vary from one migraineur to the next.

This sequence of images illustrates how some people have described their auras. Image A represents normal vision. The onset of aura in image B is a bright point of light forming within a blind spot in the visual field. As the blind spot expands in image C, the bright light evolves into a jagged crescent shape. Aura generally lasts from 10 to 25 minutes before disappearing.

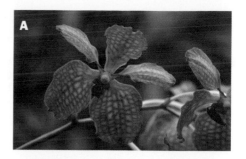

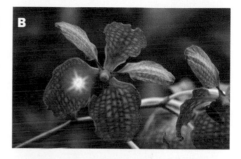

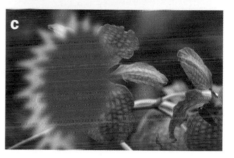

Brain response during aura

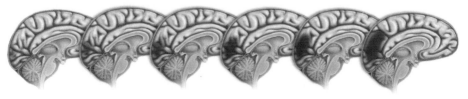

approximately 10-minute time span ⟶

This illustration represents the wave-like movement of altered activity that spreads gradually across the visual cortex of the brain during visual aura. The visual cortex is located in the occipital lobe at the back of the brain.

Cluster headache

Abnormal function of the hypothalamus

Research, using brain imaging, shows that abnormal activity takes place in the hypothalamus on the same side that the pain of cluster headache is occurring, The hypothalamus controls many vital processes, including the sleep-wake cycle and other internal rhythms.

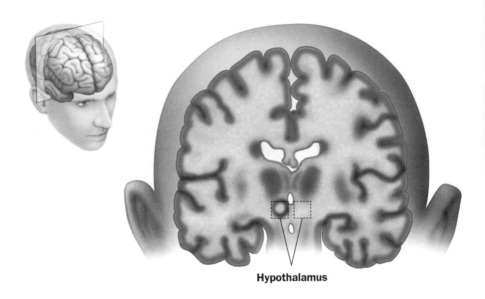

Hypothalamus

Response of the autonomic nervous system

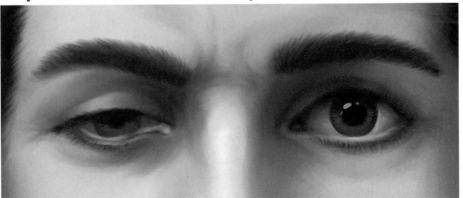

Characteristic responses of the autonomic nervous system to cluster headache are a tearing of the eye and stuffy or runny nose on the side of the head affected by the pain. The eye may be red, the size of the pupil reduced and the eyelid drooping.

Trigeminal neuralgia

Trigeminal nerve

The trigminal nerve is one of the 12 pairs of cranial nerves that supply the sense organs and muscles of the head. A cranial nerve emerges directly from the skull (cranium), as opposed to a spinal nerve that emerges from the spinal column.

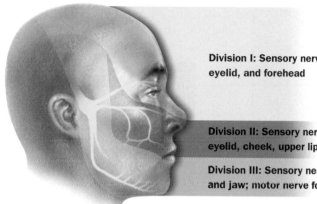

Division I: Sensory nerves for the eyeball, upper eyelid, and forehead

Division II: Sensory nerves for the nostril, lower eyelid, cheek, upper lip and upper gum

Division III: Sensory nerve for the lower gum, lower lip and jaw; motor nerve for the muscles of the jaw

Trigeminal neuralgia may occur when a blood vessel comes in direct contact with the trigeminal nerve (see inset). If medications don't provide relief, doctors may try to deaden part of the nerve or surgically relocate the blood vessel.

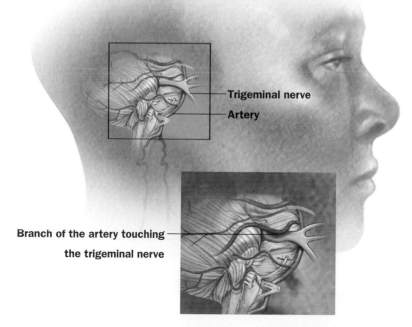

Trigeminal nerve

Artery

Branch of the artery touching the trigeminal nerve

Secondary causes of headache

Subdural hematoma

Head trauma can cause blood vessels (veins) along the brain's surface to tear. The rupture allows blood to collect beneath the dura mater (subdural) and form a mass (hematoma) that puts pressure on brain tissue, possibly resulting in a headache.

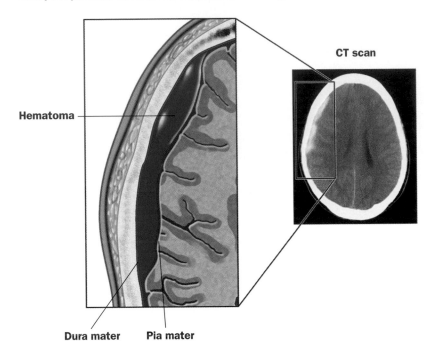

Epidural hematoma

Head trauma from a skull fracture may cause an artery to rupture between the dura mater and the skull, resulting in a hematoma and possibly a headache.

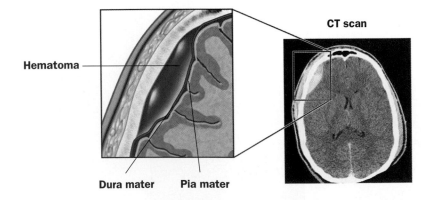

Brain tumor

Normal pressure within the brain may be altered when the abnormal growth of brain cells forms a tumor. A headache is a common, early symptom of a brain tumor. Over time, the pain typically becomes continuous and more severe. In most cases, other symptoms will accompany the headache.

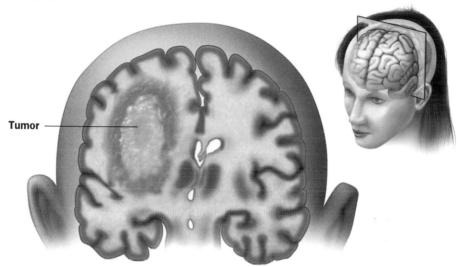

Tumor

Carotid dissection

A dissection in the wall of a carotid artery can block blood flow to the brain (below right). An early sign of this condition is often a headache. In many cases, other neurologic signs and symptoms accompany the headache.

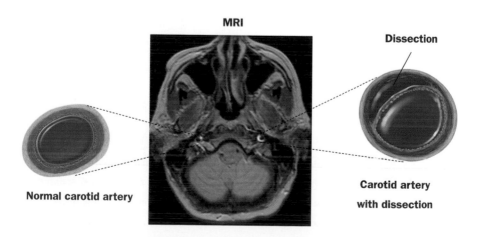

MRI

Dissection

Normal carotid artery

Carotid artery
with dissection

How triptans may work

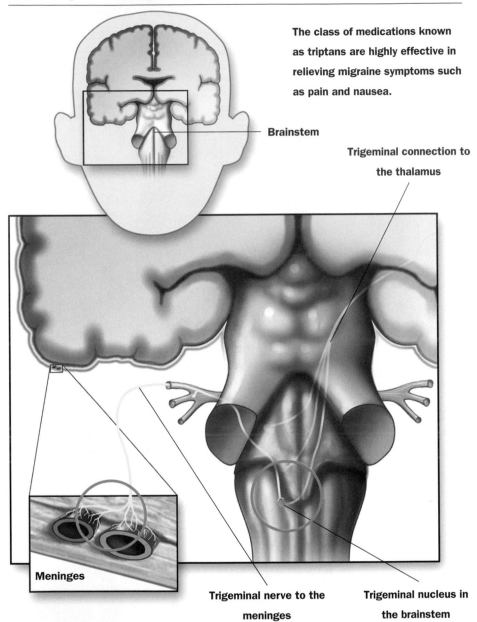

The class of medications known as triptans are highly effective in relieving migraine symptoms such as pain and nausea.

Brainstem

Trigeminal connection to the thalamus

Meninges

Trigeminal nerve to the meninges

Trigeminal nucleus in the brainstem

Triptans have their effect on migraine by attaching to subtypes of serotonin receptors. Serotonin is a brain chemical that regulates pain messages. The receptors are located on blood vessels and nerves in the meninges and on nerve cells in the trigeminal nucleus. The action of triptans may take place at these two locations (green circles), stopping migraine pain and associated symptoms.

Chapter 7

Nonmedication therapy

There's no question that headache medications offer a quick, simple response to head pain. Yet nonmedication therapies can play an important role in managing your headache and frequently supplement the effectiveness of drug therapy. Nonmedication therapies include making many healthy, positive changes to your daily routine and implementing various strategies to manage stress or to relax.

There are several reasons why you may wish to restrict or not use medications for your migraine and place greater emphasis on nonmedication options. The use of drugs may:

- Lead to rebound headaches from medication overuse
- Interfere with other medical conditions
- Cause unwanted side effects
- Be ineffective at treating your migraine
- Be unnecessary because your headache is not severe

One or more nonmedication therapies may offer you a viable alternative to medications and eliminate or lessen some of the negative effects noted above. However, nonmedication therapies often are not effective when used alone, at least for moderate or severe migraine. They may reduce headache frequency but likely won't relieve the pain. In general, nonmedication therapies are used in combination with medications for best results.

Because many nonmedication therapies involve long-term changes in your personal habits and behaviors, it's important that you talk to your doctor before you act. These seemingly straightforward measures do hold some potential risks. Your doctor can help you develop a safe program that gets the most out of your effort.

Self-care techniques

Self-care techniques for headache are practical measures that you can take to alleviate the acute symptoms of migraine, including pain, nausea and sensitivity to light and sound. They're most often used at the beginning of a headache. And they can be used at home and often outside the home.

Here are some conventional, self-care methods to treat the occasional migraine. As you read the tips, you may find that you're already using self-care without being aware of it.

Temperature therapy. Applying hot or cold compresses to sensitive areas of the head or neck may reduce headache pain. Ice packs have a numbing effect and may dull the sensation of pain. Hot packs and heating pads can relax tense muscles and increase blood flow. Warm showers or baths may have a similar effect.

Massage. Applying gentle pressure to affected areas may temporarily reduce the severity of head pain. Having someone give you a brief shoulder or neck massage may also alleviate muscle tension that's contributing to your migraine.

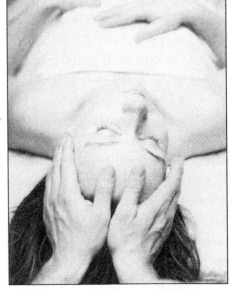

Calming environment. You may find that you're sensitive to light or sound when experiencing a migraine. Sitting or lying in a dark, quiet room may reduce the pain and help you relax. Sleep may also help ease the attack.

Behavior therapy

Behavior therapy works in two important ways. It encourages you to (1) change behavior that makes your headaches worse and (2) reinforce behavior that makes your headaches better. This approach may require you to modify your emotional reactions to pain and other symptoms of migraine. It often involves adjusting your daily routine and making small changes in your lifestyle. With behavior therapy, you may better understand your condition, learn to evaluate priorities and cope with headache more effectively.

Behavioral techniques are used primarily as preventive measures. Commonly used strategies include lifestyle changes, stress management therapy and relaxation training. Each therapy, described separately below, may be used alone or in combination with medications or other nonmedication therapies.

Lifestyle changes

Long-term headache prevention may require you to identify factors that prompt a migraine — factors known as headache triggers. With the help of a headache diary, you may begin to notice patterns in your daily life that correspond with your migraine attacks. Maybe you notice that you always get a headache after drinking a glass of red wine. Or perhaps your headache occurs at times when you've had little sleep. It could be that patterns of sleep, diet and exercise trigger your migraine.

Sleep patterns
Sleep refreshes you and gives you energy for doing physical activity and for fighting off fatigue and stress. It also boosts your immune system, reducing your risk of illness. But if you're like many people with migraine, you may find that head pain keeps you from falling asleep or that it wakes you up at night.

You may also find that your headache is triggered by a poor night's sleep. Often, this is a result of stress, too much caffeine, alcohol consumption or an improper diet. There also may be a rela-

To nap, or not to nap?

The urge for a midday snooze is built into your body's biological clock. It generally occurs between 1 p.m. and 4 p.m., when your body temperature is programmed to dip slightly. Napping isn't a substitute for a full night's sleep. But if a nap refreshes you and doesn't interfere with nighttime sleep, you may follow these guidelines:

Keep the nap short. Thirty minutes is ideal. Naps longer than one hour are more likely to interfere with your nighttime sleep.

Take a mid-afternoon nap. Naps at this time of day usually produce a more restful slumber.

Rest a bit. If you can't nap, you can still lie down for a few minutes with your eyes closed and focus your mind on something calming.

tionship between your headache and sleep disorders such as obstructive sleep apnea, in which the air passages of the upper respiratory tract are repeatedly obstructed while you sleep.

It's important to get adequate rest. About eight hours is sufficient for most people. While that may seem easier said than done, there are ways to prepare for sleep. Here are strategies that may help you take advantage of available sleep time:

Relax before bedtime. This may include simple things such as having a light snack, listening to soothing music, taking a warm bath or reading. The idea is to unwind so that you won't take stress and worry to bed with you.

Establish regular sleep hours. Try going to bed and waking up at the same time each day, even on weekends. A regular pattern often improves sleep.

Don't try to sleep. The harder you try to sleep, the more awake you'll feel. Read or watch television until you become drowsy and fall asleep naturally.

Watch what you eat and drink before bedtime. A light snack may help you relax before sleeping. However, avoid heavy meals since they could cause heartburn or irritate your esophagus. Caffeine, nicotine and alcohol can also delay sleep.

Minimize distractions. Save your bedroom for sleep or intimacy. Don't watch television or take work materials to bed. Close your bedroom door or create a subtle background noise, with the use of a fan, for example, to muffle distracting noises. Drink less before bed so that you won't have to go to the bathroom at night.

Check your medications. Ask your doctor if your prescription drugs may be contributing to sleep problems. Check any over-the-counter products to see if they contain caffeine or other stimulants, such as pseudoephedrine. This is especially important to do for migraine medications, which often contain caffeine.

Diet

A nutritious diet plays a major role in good health, even in preventing migraine. Hunger — from skipping meals, not eating enough, dieting or fasting — can be a migraine trigger for some people. In addition, certain foods may trigger a migraine (see Chapter 4 for more details). By avoiding triggers, you may reduce the number of migraine attacks.

This doesn't mean you remove all foods from your diet that you've heard are potential triggers. Food that may cause a headache in one person may not affect another. The best way to identify a food trigger is through a careful process of elimination. Your headache diary will be very helpful in this process. If you suspect that a certain food is a trigger, eliminate this food — and only this food — from your diet for a period of time, at least for the interval of time you normally have between headaches. Does this appear to reduce the frequency of your migraine attacks? If so, slowly add the potential trig-

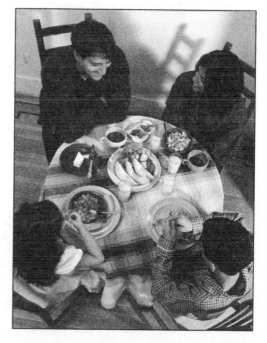

ger back into your diet. If you have an attack after reintroducing the food, remove it again. This food may indeed be considered a migraine trigger. You should go through this process, one food at a time, for each food you think might be a culprit.

A pattern between your eating habits and your migraine attacks may indicate a food trigger, but it may also be just a coincidence. Food triggers can be difficult to detect, even after a lengthy trial-and-error process. Many people aren't able to identify triggers with any certainty.

Here are commonsense tips for dealing with migraine that may be related to diet and food triggers:

Establish a regular eating schedule. A regular schedule means eating at about the same time everyday and not skipping meals, especially breakfast. Almost half of the people who get headaches report that fasting will trigger their condition.

Avoid headache triggers, but don't let this cause you stress. If you spend too much time and energy worrying about food triggers, it may result in a stress-induced headache.

Eat foods rich in magnesium. An estimated 50 percent of people with migraine may have a magnesium deficiency. Magnesium is abundant in nuts, legumes, dark green leafy vegetables, and whole-grain cereals and breads.

Caffeine as a cure?

Caffeine can help relieve a headache, and it can cause a headache, too. Some people have found that drinking a cup of coffee or a soda containing caffeine may actually reduce head pain.

Caffeine is a mild stimulant and, in small amounts, can enhance the pain-reducing effects of acetaminophen and aspirin. However, when you drink caffeine frequently and then don't consume it for a while, you may get a headache as the result of withdrawal.

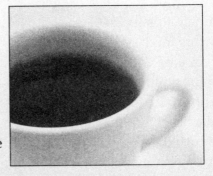

Exercise habits

Regular exercise can help reduce migraine pain. During physical activity, your body releases certain chemicals that block pain signals to your brain. These chemicals also help alleviate anxiety and depression, conditions that can exacerbate pain.

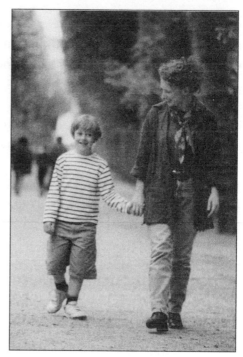

Studies indicate that when inactive people begin aerobic exercise, such as walking or running, for 30 minutes a day three days a week, the average frequency of headaches drops by 50 percent or more after several weeks. If your doctor agrees, choose any exercise you enjoy, including walking, swimming or cycling. Your doctor can also advise you about the potential side effects of combining certain migraine medications with exercise.

Exercise also may trigger a migraine attack. This is often a result of too vigorous exercise for your level of fitness — for example, if you're really out of shape before you start exercising or you increase the intensity of your workout too quickly. Start slowly and at a comfortable pace. Once you're able to successfully exercise at a low intensity on a regular basis, you may want to increase gradually to a more moderate workout. It may help to take an analgesic about 20 minutes before you begin exercising, as long as you do so in moderation and with your doctor's approval.

Stress prevention and management

Pain and stress seem to go hand in hand. When you're in pain from a migraine, minor hassles turn into major obstacles. Common signs and symptoms of stress include anxiety and irritability, changes in eating or sleep patterns, and increased alcohol or drug abuse. Stress may also cause you to do things that intensify pain, such as tensing your muscles, gritting your teeth and stiffening your shoulders.

A first step in breaking the pain-stress cycle is to realize that stress is your response to an event, not the event itself. It's something you can try to control. By reducing stress, you may likely experience less frequent and less intense migraine.

Identifying causes of stress

Take some time to think about what causes stress in your life. Stress may be linked to external factors, such as family, work, finances and unpredictable events. Stress can also come from within. Negative attitudes, unrealistic expectations and poor health habits are internal factors that can cause stress.

Now ask yourself if there's anything you can do to avoid these sources of stress or lessen their impact. There are some situations you can control and some you can't. Concentrate on the situations you can control or change. For situations that are beyond your control, look for ways to remain calm under trying circumstances.

Strategies for reducing stress

It's one thing to be aware of stress in your daily life, but it's another to know how to reduce it. As you consider your list of stressors (the things that cause you stress), think about why they're problems for you. Then consider how you can reduce their impact.

Plan your day. Planning ahead can help you feel more in control of your life. You might start by getting up 15 minutes earlier to ease the morning rush. Organize your daily activities so that you're not faced with scheduling conflicts or last-minute rushes. Do difficult or unpleasant tasks early in the day and be done with them. Try to keep your plan flexible because a migraine can happen at any time and you may need to change course.

Simplify your schedule. Prioritize your tasks and accomplish them at a pace you can handle. Learn to delegate responsibility to others and say no to added commitments if you're not up to doing them. Try not to feel guilty if you aren't productive every waking moment. Take time to relax or stretch periodically during the day.

Get organized. Organize your workspace at home and on the job so that you know where things are. Keep appliances and accessories in working order to prevent untimely repairs.

Change the pace. Occasionally break away from your routine and try something new. Take a vacation, even if it's just a weekend getaway. A change of pace can help develop a new outlook.

Deal with your anger. Anger needs to be expressed, but carefully. Count to 10, and use that time to compose yourself. Then you can convey your anger in a more effective manner.

Be positive. Avoid negative self-talk. Try to convince yourself that there's no room for "Yes, but . . . ." Also, it helps to spend time with people who have a positive outlook and a sense of humor. Laughter actually helps ease pain.

Be patient. Don't expect too much too soon. Be aware that improvements to your health may take time.

Let others help. Recognize when you need the support of family and friends. Talking about your problems with others can often relieve pent-up emotions and lead to solutions you hadn't thought of on your own.

Relaxation techniques

You can't avoid all sources of stress. But you can change how you react to stress. Relaxation can help you reduce anxiety, increase your self-control and remain alert and productive. Keep in mind, though, that the benefits of relaxation are only as good as your efforts to relax. Learning to relax takes time.

Breathing exercises

If you're like most adults, you breathe from your chest. Breathing exercises, then, will require you to relearn something you did naturally as a child. Children generally breathe from their diaphragm, the muscle that separates the chest from the abdomen. Deep breathing from your diaphragm is more relaxing than breathing from higher in your chest. Try to do 20 minutes of deep breathing every day for good health, not just when you're stressed.

Here's an exercise to help you learn to do deep, relaxed breathing. Practice it until it becomes natural.

- Lie down on your back or sit comfortably with your feet flat on the floor.
- Rest one hand on your abdomen and one hand on your chest. This will allow you to feel the natural movements of your breathing and thus help you control the exercise better.
- Inhale while pushing the muscles in your abdomen out. You may breathe through your nose or your mouth.
- Slowly exhale while gently relaxing your abdomen. Make each breath a smooth, wave-like motion.
- Pause for a moment. Then repeat this exercise for one to two minutes, until you feel better. If you experience lightheadedness, shorten the length or depth of your breathing.

Biofeedback

Biofeedback is a procedure in which a therapist uses monitoring instruments to help teach you how to control bodily responses that can affect your health. The initial sessions may be performed in a physical therapy clinic or medical center, where you practice this technique so you can use it in your own home. According to a 1995 consensus statement from the National Institutes of Health, there is evidence that biofeedback can help to relieve types of chronic pain, including migraine, as well as ease the effects of conditions such as asthma and high blood pressure.

To learn this technique, a biofeedback therapist applies sensors to various parts of your body. The sensors help track your responses and give you auditory or visual feedback. For example, you might see a monitor that displays your levels of muscle tension, brain wave activity, heart rate, blood pressure, breathing rate or skin temperature.

Tips for relaxation success

If relaxation is new to you, you may not notice immediate ben-fits. Work on your relaxation skills at least once or twice a day until they come naturally. A quiet place and a recording of relaxing music or sounds often help.

Get comfortable. Loosen tight clothing and remove your shoes and belt, if need be.

Vary your practice times. Practice relaxation at different times throughout the day. The idea is to learn how to relax whenever you need to.

Stay focused. It's normal for your mind to wander and dwell on demands of the day when you start out with these exercises. Just keep focusing your attention back on relaxation.

Enjoy the moment. When you're finished, sit quietly for a minute or two to make the transition back to the real world.

With this feedback, you can learn how to produce changes inter-nally that promote relaxation and help you cope with stress. After training, many people can use the principles of biofeedback at home to ease a slow-forming migraine attack. Thermal biofeedback, the preferred method for migraine, focuses on skin temperature. By concentrating on raising your skin temperature, you can help ease migraine pain.

Progressive muscle relaxation

A commonly used relaxation strategy for headache is progressive muscle relaxation. This technique involves working with different muscle groups, one group at a time. You first raise the tension level in a muscle group, such as in a leg or an arm, by tightening the muscles. Then you relax and let the tension go. Move on progres-sively to each muscle group. Be careful, however, not to tightly tense muscles in your face or neck, as this may trigger pain.

By the time you have gone through all the muscle groups, your body should feel less tense. With repeated practice, you may be able to relax muscles quickly and deeply, even in stressful situa-tions that tend to trigger migraine.

Both biofeedback and progressive muscle relaxation training have been shown to lessen headache severity and frequency by 45 percent to 60 percent. This is about the same success rate as some headache medications, but without any side effects.

Seeking help with nonmedication therapies

You may find that nonmedication therapies are difficult for you to stick with. Long-term lifestyle changes can be hard to maintain. After a while, you may find yourself back in the pattern of sleeping late on weekends or skipping exercise. If you struggle with making a permanent change, try to find a friend or family member who is willing to exercise or attend sessions with you. Explain to others about your need to keep a regular schedule. You may be surprised by how supportive those around you can be if they understand what you're experiencing. All of these efforts will help you receive the full benefits of a valuable component of your headache management plan and reduce your dependence on medications.

Part 3

Other types of headache

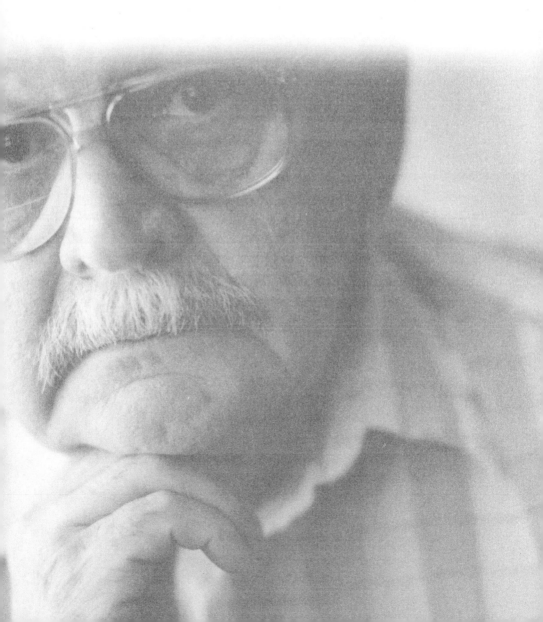

Chapter 8

Tension-type headache

Picture in your mind a stressed-out office worker swallowed up by paper piles stacked to the ceiling, or a harried parent escorting kids across town from one activity to another. If, as the saying goes, "a picture is worth a thousand words," either of these situations depicts a tension-type headache about to happen. Imagine yourself as the main character in the picture and you can almost feel the kind of headache that's about to follow — a band of aching pressure encompassing your head.

Tension-type headache is the most common headache, and yet it's one of the least understood. Experts continue to debate its causes and even its name. Over the years, as different theories emerged about the origins of this type of headache, it was known by names such as muscle contraction headache, psychogenic headache, depressive headache, essential headache and ordinary headache.

One prevalent theory was that chronic tension in the scalp, neck and jaw muscles caused this type of head pain. Thus, it became known as a tension headache. But many researchers began to question this idea. As a result, the International Headache Society settled on the term *tension-type headache*, reflecting the fact that muscle tension is associated with this kind of head pain but doesn't seem to be a main cause. The pain appears to have other triggers or may be a result of no apparent cause.

A common condition

No matter what you call it, tension-type headache probably accounts for a majority of all primary headaches. And it's more common in women than in men. Up to 88 percent of women and 69 percent of men experience tension-type headaches during their life-times. Tension-type headache is most prevalent in people between the ages of 30 and 39. After age 39, prevalence declines. The majori-ty of people who get migraine also get tension-type pain.

Because tension-type headache is so common, its impact on job productivity and overall quality of life is considerable. When your head is "gripped in a vise," as the pain is often described, you may feel unable to attend family and social activities. You might need to stay home from work, or if you do go to your job, you work at only a fraction of your normal efficiency.

Few people with this type of headache seek medical attention. One reason is that tension-type headache usually is easy to treat with over-the-counter medications. Other reasons may be a fear of not being taken seriously by the doctor or the misperception that tension-type headache is purely psychological in nature — that admitting you have one means you're weak or neurotic.

While much remains unknown and even controversial about tension-type headache, this condition is widely recognized as a bio-logic disorder. And fortunately, while doctors may disagree about what causes this type of headache, they do know how to help you. Many medications can provide fast and effective pain relief.

Signs and symptoms

Tension-type headache usually produces a dull, achy pain or sensa-tion of tightness in your forehead or at the sides and back of your head. Many people liken the feeling to having a tight band of pres-sure encircling their heads. In its most extensive form, the pain feels like a hooded cape that drapes down over the shoulders.

The headache is usually described as mild to moderately intense. The severity of the pain varies from one person to another, and from one headache to another in the same person. One attack of a tension-type headache can last from 30 minutes to an entire week. Most people report that the pain starts soon after waking in the morning or early in the day.

Some people with tension-type headache experience neck or jaw discomfort or a clicking sound when opening the jaw. There may also be tenderness on the scalp, neck and shoulder muscles. Other signs and symptoms may include difficulty sleeping, fatigue, irritability, loss of appetite and difficulty concentrating.

Unlike some forms of migraine, tension-type headache usually isn't associated with visual disturbances (blind spots or flashing lights), nausea, vomiting, abdominal pain, weakness or numbness on one side of the body, or slurred speech. While physical activity typically aggravates migraine pain, it doesn't make tension-type headache pain any worse. A few people with tension-type headache will experience an increased sensitivity to light or sound, but this isn't a common symptom.

Triggers and aggravators

The list of possible triggers of tension-type headache is a long one. You may have no identifiable or consistent trigger, or have several obvious ones. The potential triggers include:

- Stress
- Depression and anxiety
- Lack of sleep or changes in sleep routine
- Skipping meals
- Poor posture
- Working in awkward positions or holding one position for a long time
- Lack of physical activity
- Occasionally, hormonal changes related to menstruation, pregnancy, menopause or hormone use
- Medications used for other conditions, such as depression or high blood pressure
- Overuse of headache medication

Stress is the most common trigger reported for tension-type headache. Studies show that among groups of people who may share similar kinds of stressful life events, the people with tension-type headache are more likely to perceive such events negatively and have less effective coping strategies.

Tension-type headache may be made worse by jaw pain from clenching or grinding teeth or by head trauma, such as a blow to the head or whiplash injury. People with stiff joints and muscles due to arthritis of the neck or inflammation of the shoulder joints may develop tension-type headache.

Causes

The exact cause or causes of tension-type headache are unknown. Different theories have been proposed about the mechanism underlying this type of head pain. Until a few years ago, many researchers believed that the pain of tension-type headache stemmed from muscle contraction in the face, neck and scalp, perhaps as a result of heightened emotions, tension or stress.

More recent research discredits this theory. Studies using a test called an electromyogram, which records the electric currents generated by muscle activity, haven't detected increased muscle tension in people diagnosed with tension-type headache. Not only that, but people with migraine have as much if not more muscle tension than people with tension-type headache.

Researchers now believe that tension-type headache may result from changes among certain brain chemicals — serotonin, endorphins and numerous other chemicals — that help nerves communicate. These are similar biochemical changes associated with migraine. Although it's not clear why the chemical levels fluctuate, the process is thought to activate pain pathways to the brain and to interfere with the brain's ability to suppress the pain. On one hand, tight muscles in the neck and scalp may contribute to a headache in someone with altered chemical levels. On the other hand, the tight muscles may be a result of these chemical changes.

Another chemical in the body that may play a role in tension-type headache is nitric oxide, which is involved in the transmission of nerve impulses. Overproduction of nitric oxide has been linked to chronic tension-type headache and migraine. And substances that block the production of nitric oxide have been shown to reduce the muscle tightness associated with tension-type headache.

Because both tension-type headache and migraine involve similar changes in brain chemicals, some researchers believe that the two types of headache are related. A majority of people diagnosed as having migraine also get occasional tension-type headache, and a quarter of people diagnosed with tension-type headache get occasional migraine. Some experts speculate that migraine may develop from the regular occurrence of tension-type headache. The distinctive migraine features form as the pain becomes more severe. Other research suggests that mild migraine is in reality a type of tension-type headache.

Types

Tension-type headache is classified into two forms — episodic and chronic. This classification distinguishes between occasional headaches separated by varying lengths of time between attacks and frequent headaches that occur, in many cases, almost daily.

Episodic
Episodic tension-type headache occurs on fewer than 15 days a month. These headaches are usually brief, lasting a few minutes to a few hours. In one survey of people with episodic tension-type headache, 63 percent had scalp and neck muscle tenderness in addition to head pain. People with increasingly frequent attacks of the episodic form may be at higher risk of developing the chronic form of the headache over a period of years.

Chronic
Chronic tension-type headache occurs on 15 days a month or more for at least three months. Compared with the episodic form, chronic tension-type headache is less common, but twice as many women as men have the chronic form. The duration and the severity of episodic and chronic tension-type headaches are similar, although

> ### Depression, anxiety and chronic tension-type headache
>
> People with chronic tension-type headache are more likely to experience anxiety or depression, compared with people who don't have headaches. Whether these mood disorders contribute to the headaches or vice versa is uncertain — it's a bit like asking which came first, the chicken or the egg.
>
> Many people who have tension-type headache say the pain often occurs during or after times of heightened stress and anxiety. If you do have a mood disorder, it's critical to treat this condition as well as your headache to achieve the best possible outcome. For example, if you have both depression and tension-type headache, treatment for your headaches may be less effective if the depression goes undiagnosed and untreated.

for many people with the chronic form, pain is daily and almost continuous. Like the episodic form, chronic tension-type headache can be with or without scalp tenderness.

People whose parents, siblings or children have chronic tension-type headache are three times as likely to develop the chronic form themselves. Although this suggests a genetic predisposition, it's unlikely that a single "headache gene" is responsible. More likely, multiple factors, including an inherited susceptibility, play a role.

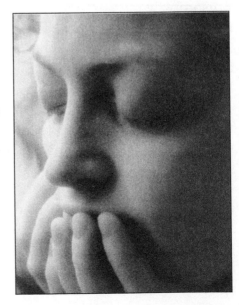

Controversy surrounds the issue of whether chronic tension-type headache is really a separate entity from chronic migraine. Doctors often have trouble distinguishing between the two types of headache. Both disorders are thought to stem from episodic headaches after pain pathways become sensitized, and both involve similar biochemical changes in the brain.

Treatment

Most people don't consult a doctor for help in dealing with occasional attacks of tension-type headache. For many, a couple of over-the-counter pain relievers, a few moments to relax and a good night's sleep provide enough relief. Others may seek help if their headaches occur frequently or the pain is severe.

If tension-type headache disrupts your life, don't hesitate to talk to your doctor. The condition is a biological disorder that can be treated effectively. A comprehensive approach, involving both non-medication and medication therapies, is successful for more than 90 percent of people with tension-type headache who seek assistance.

Nonmedication therapy

Rest, ice packs or a long, hot shower may be all you need to relieve a tension-type headache. As discussed in Chapter 7, a variety of nonmedication strategies can help reduce the severity and frequency of chronic headache. This approach can be a vital part of any treatment plan for headache.

Healthy lifestyle. Behaviors that promote general good health also may help prevent headache. These lifestyle measures include following regular eating and sleeping schedules and avoiding excess caffeine. It's also important to stay physically active. Regular aerobic exercise, such as walking, swimming or biking, can help reduce the frequency of tension-type headache. If you already have a headache, exercise may help relieve the pain. But be sure to talk to your doctor before starting any exercise program.

Stress management. Stress is the most commonly reported trigger for tension-type headache. One way to help reduce stress is by planning ahead and organizing your day. Another way is to allow more time to relax. And if you're caught in a stressful situation, consider stepping back and allowing emotions to settle.

A variety of relaxation techniques are useful in coping with tension-type headache, including deep breathing and biofeedback (see Chapter 7 for details on the various techniques). If anxiety or depression is an issue, behavior therapy may be helpful for dealing with stress and pain.

Muscle relaxation. Muscle tension is associated with tension-type headache. Applying heat or ice to sore muscles may ease the tension. Which treatment to apply is a matter of personal preference — some people find heat more effective, while others prefer cold. If heat is your choice, you may use a heating pad set on low, a hot-water bottle, a warm compress or a hot towel. A hot bath or shower also may help. If cold is your choice, wrap the ice pack in a cloth before use to protect your skin.

Massage is a wonderful way to relieve muscle tension. For some people, it also may provide relief from headache pain. Gently massage the muscles of your head, neck and shoulders with your fingertips. Or have someone else do the massage for you.

Perfecting your posture

Good posture can help keep your muscles from tensing up. It places minimal strain on your muscles, ligaments, tendons and bones. Good posture supports and protects all parts of your body and allows you to move efficiently. When standing, hold your shoulders back and your head high. Pull in your abdomen and buttocks and tuck in your chin. When sitting, make sure your thighs are parallel to the ground and your head isn't slumped forward.

Try to avoid sitting, standing or working in one position for long periods of time. Wearing poorly fitting shoes or high heels also can cause posture problems. Do regular stretching and strengthening exercises for your neck and shoulders. Here are other tips for improving your posture:

- Stand with your weight on both feet.
- When standing in one place, put one foot up on a stool or chair rung and switch to the other foot periodically.
- Don't carry a shoulder bag that weighs more than two pounds.
- Sit in a straight-back chair with your back supported.
- When sitting for long periods, occasionally elevate your legs by placing your feet on a footstool. If possible, get up and move around every half-hour or so.

Medication therapy

A variety of medications, both over-the-counter (OTC) and pre-scription, are available for treating tension-type headache. Many people find fast, effective relief by taking pain relievers such as aspirin, ibuprofen (Advil, Motrin, others) or acetaminophen (Tylenol, others). These medications are inexpensive and readily available and don't require a prescription from your doctor.

People with severe or chronic tension-type headache may re-quire stronger painkillers or preventive medications to reduce the frequency and severity of head pain. Which drug works best varies from one person to another.

Whether you have episodic or chronic headaches, it's important not to overuse OTC medications — limit your use of painkillers to two days a week. Try to take the medications only when necessary, and use the smallest dose needed to relieve your pain. Overusing pain medications can cause rebound headaches or the development of chronic daily headache (see Chapter 9), triggering the very symptoms you're trying to stop. In addition, all medications used to treat headache have side effects, some of which may be serious. For prescription medications, of course, follow the recommended dosage and do not exceed it.

Acute therapy. Acute therapy aims to stop or reduce the pain of an existing headache attack. Many different medications are used for the acute treatment of tension-type headache:

Analgesics. Analgesics are pain relievers. Acetaminophen (Tylenol, others) and a class of drugs known nonsteroidal anti-inflammatory drugs (NSAIDs) are effective in reducing headache pain. Side effects of acetaminophen are extremely rare but if the drug is taken in large doses for long periods of time, it can cause serious liver damage. NSAIDs include the OTC drugs aspirin, ibuprofen (Advil, Motrin, others) and naproxen sodium (Aleve, Anaprox). Prescription NSAIDs include naproxen (Naprelan, Naprosyn), ketoprofen (Orudis), indomethacin (Indocin) and ketorolac tromethamine (Toradol). Side effects include nausea, diar-rhea or constipation, stomach or abdominal pain, stomach bleeding, and ulcers. You can reduce or eliminate these symptoms by taking NSAIDs after meals or with milk.

A group of NSAIDs known as cyclooxygenase-2 (COX-2) inhibitors, including celecoxib (Celebrex), rofecoxib (Vioxx) and valdecoxib (Bextra), offer effective pain relief with less likelihood of stomach irritation and other gastrointestinal symptoms. Although they show promise, it should be noted that COX-2 inhibitors haven't been studied specifically for the treatment of headache.

Combination medications. Aspirin or acetaminophen (or both of these analgesics) is often combined with caffeine or a sedative drug, such as butalbital, in a single medication. For example, Excedrin combines aspirin, acetaminophen and caffeine. Combination drugs such as this may be more effective than are pure analgesics for pain relief. Also, brand name drugs such as Amidrine, Midrin and Migrex are analgesic, sedative and vasoconstrictor combinations that sometimes are used to treat tension-type headache.

Although many combination drugs are available over the counter, analgesic-sedative combinations can be obtained only by prescription because they may be addictive and can lead to chronic daily headache. They should be used no more than one day a week and their use carefully monitored by a physician.

Other medications. For people who experience both migraine and episodic tension-type headache, a triptan can effectively relieve the pain of both headaches. Opiates, or narcotics, are rarely used because of their side effects and potential for dependency. They include codeine combined with acetaminophen (Tylenol With Codeine No. 3) and oxycodone (OxyContin, Roxicodone).

Preventive therapy. Preventive medication is taken at regular intervals to reduce the frequency and severity of attacks. The medication may be prescribed for people who have more than two headaches a week or who have tension-type headache that isn't relieved by acute medication and nondrug therapy. Your doctor also may recommend preventive medication if your headache lasts longer than three to four hours, if severe pain becomes disabling or causes you to overuse acute medication, or if you can't take acute medication because of other medical conditions.

Antidepressants are often used to prevent tension-type headache, especially the chronic form. These drugs aren't painkillers. Rather, they work to stabilize the levels of brain chemicals such as serotonin, which may be involved in the development of a head-ache. You don't have to have depression in order to use these drugs. NSAIDs, muscle relaxants and migraine medications also may be used to prevent tension-type headache.

Tricyclic antidepressants. This group of antidepressants, includ-ing amitriptyline (Elavil) and nortriptyline (Aventyl, Pamelor), are the most commonly used medications to prevent tension-type headache. They're effective against both the episodic and chronic forms. Side effects of these medications may include weight gain, drowsiness, dry mouth, blurred vision and constipation. Older adults also may experience confusion or faintness when taking tri-cyclic antidepressants.

Selective serotonin reuptake inhibitors (SSRIs). Antidepressants such as paroxetine (Paxil), venlafaxine (Effexor) and fluoxetine (Prozac, Sarafem) produce fewer side effects than do the tricyclic antidepressants but generally are less reliable in preventing headache. Further studies are needed to demonstrate their effec-tiveness.

NSAIDs. Chronic tension-type headache may be effectively managed with NSAIDs such as ibuprofen and ketoprofen. In these circumstances, the medication is taken daily.

Other medications. Medications that may be used to prevent tension-type headache include divalproex (Depakote) and gaba-pentin (Neurontin). Both drugs were developed to treat seizure dis-orders but sometimes can prevent headache. Muscle relaxants such as tizanidine (Zanaflex) also have been effective. Migraine medica-tions sometimes are used to prevent tension-type headache, al-though few studies indicate how effective they are. Studies on an experimental drug that blocks the production of nitric oxide in the brain show it to be effective in reducing headache pain.

Preventive medications usually require several weeks to build up in the nervous system before they take effect. So don't get frus-trated if you haven't seen improvements shortly after starting the drug — it may take a couple of months or longer. A combination of different medications may be needed for maximum effectiveness. Also be aware that overusing caffeine or painkillers for acute relief may reduce the effect of a preventive drug.

Preventive medication is considered successful if it results in a 50 percent reduction in the intensity of tension-type head pain or in the frequency and duration of attacks. To obtain the greatest benefit from preventive medication, you should limit your use of acute pain relievers to a minimum.

Your doctor will monitor your treatment to see how the preventive medication is working. If your headaches are under control, your dose of medication may be reduced gradually over time.

A balancing act

Tension-type headache can zap your productivity and stifle your social life. Fortunately, effective treatment is available if you need it. Managing tension-type headache is often a balance between fostering healthy habits, finding effective nondrug treatments and using medications appropriately.

As researchers continue to gain a better understanding of the causes of tension-type headache, their efforts may contribute to the development of new acute and preventive strategies.

Chapter 9

Chronic daily headache

As the name implies, the most striking feature of chronic daily headache is its frequency. The term actually refers to several different types of headaches that share a common characteristic of occurring several hours a day nearly every day.

Chronic daily headache, or CDH, is a common disorder, affecting nearly 5 percent of the U.S. population. It's also one of the most disabling headaches and can place an enormous burden on you and your family and friends. People with CDH commonly experience depression, anxiety, sleep disturbances, and other psychological and physical problems. Chronic headaches with this incessancy are a challenge to doctors trying to treat the condition.

To cope with the constant pain, many people with chronic daily headache depend heavily on pain medication. Ironically, heavy usage often creates what's known as rebound headaches, a cycle of frequent headaches that's hard to break.

A wide range of treatment strategies for CDH focuses on prevention. Acute treatment, which provides immediate relief of symptoms, is limited in order to avoid the rebound headaches.

With aggressive treatment initially and steady, long-term management, many people with CDH experience less head pain and fewer headaches. They see major improvements in their quality of life as the pain, depression and sleep disturbances diminish.

Classification

Chronic daily headache is an umbrella term that encompasses several headache disorders that may or may not be related to each other. Thus, the causes, signs and symptoms, and treatments for each type of headache may vary considerably. The only common feature of all types of CDH is that the headaches occur more than 15 days a month, often on a daily basis.

Doctors classify chronic daily headache into primary and secondary forms. Primary CDH often develops in people who have had migraine or tension-type headache for many years. Over time, these headaches gradually increase in frequency until they become almost daily. Secondary CDH means that an underlying disease or condition, such as meningitis, brain tumor and high blood pressure, is causing the frequent headaches.

Headache specialists further classify primary CDH into two categories — those of long duration, lasting four hours or longer, and those of shorter duration. This chapter discusses the headaches of long duration, including chronic daily headache in migraine, chronic tension-type headache, new daily persistent headache and hemicrania continua. The International Headache Society included separate entries for these headaches in their classification system rather than group them together as a distinct category.

Chronic daily headaches of short duration — those lasting less than four hours — are discussed in Chapter 10. They include cluster headache, paroxysmal hemicrania and a form of headache best known by the abbreviation SUNCT. The short-duration headaches merit discussion in a separate chapter due to distinct qualities from the long-duration forms of CDH.

Causes

The causes of chronic daily headache are not well understood. The different types of CDH may stem from different mechanisms or combination of mechanisms but ultimately, in all forms, the brain becomes overly sensitive to signals from pain-sensitive structures both inside and outside the brain. Possible mechanisms involved in the development of CDH include:

- Abnormal response of the brain to stimulation such as muscle tension or tissue inflammation
- Abnormal function of brain structures that suppress pain
- Changes in the nervous system resulting from frequent headache attacks
- Stimulation of the central nervous system due to stress, infection or trauma
- Medication overuse
- Genetic predisposition to pain sensitivity
- Injury to or painful stimulation of the upper spine

Some studies suggest that risk factors for CDH include anxiety, depression, sleep disturbances, obesity, snoring, caffeine use and episodic headaches that start coming in greater frequency. The condition is more common in women than in men.

Types

Chronic daily headache of long duration includes four major types, characterized by different signs and symptoms. The two most common types are chronic daily headache (CDH) in migraine and chronic tension-type headache (CTTH).

It can be difficult sometimes for doctors to distinguish between CDH in migraine and chronic tension-type headache. Some scientists believe that both disorders involve similar biochemical mechanisms. The day-to-day pain of both headaches can be of similar intensity, although the pain of CTTH is rarely if ever completely disabling. In addition, CTTH isn't accompanied by nausea or sensitivity to light, sound or movement — these are characteristics of migraine. Some people with a mild form of CDH in migraine, however, may have attacks that are virtually indistinguishable from attacks of chronic tension-type headache. Other people get both CDH in migraine and CTTH. Despite the ongoing debate about how to classify the different types of chronic daily headache, doctors do agree on various ways to reduce the pain.

Chronic daily headache in migraine

Individuals with episodic migraine may develop chronic daily headache years after the migraine started. Gradually, the headaches become more frequent until you experience pain nearly every day. This development is called transformed migraine.

As the headaches become more frequent, the daily pain tends to be less severe than what you were accustomed to. The common migraine symptoms of nausea and sensitivity to light and sound often diminsh. Pain may be on one or both sides of your head and may also affect your neck and face.

Unfortunately, many people who develop transformed migraine continue to have acute migraine attacks, which are more severe than the steady, low-grade pain of the daily attacks. Both the acute and chronic forms of migraine may have the same triggers, such as alcohol, changes in sleep patterns, skipping meals, weather changes, menstruation or stress.

For people who seek medical care for transformed migraine, medication overuse is often found to be responsible. Their headaches revert to an episodic pattern within eight weeks of stopping the overuse of analgesic drugs. The International Classification of Headache Disorders also includes criteria for the diagnosis of a condition known as chronic migraine, which requires the appearance of migraine on 15 days or more a month, in the absence of medication overuse. This condition is relatively uncommon.

Many people with chronic daily headache in migraine also have depression. The depression may lift when the cycle of medication overuse and severe daily headache is broken. Chronic daily headache also is associated with sleep disturbances, anxiety, panic, irritable bowel syndrome and fibromyalgia.

Chronic tension-type headache

The characteristics of chronic tension-type headache (CTTH) are similar to those of the episodic form, but attacks occur almost every day. The signs and symptoms of tension-type headache are described in Chapter 8. The progression of occasional tension-type headaches into daily headaches can happen spontaneously or as a result of the overuse of pain medications.

The pain of CTTH is mild or moderately intense. It often involves both sides of the head and the back of the head and neck. It may feel like tightness, a bursting sensation or a dull ache — often described as a tight band of pressure around the head. The pain may fluctuate throughout the day or be steady for days, weeks or even years at a time. CTTH isn't associated with nausea or sensitivity to light or sound.

New daily persistent headache

The unique feature of this rare type of headache is its abrupt onset in people who have had no history of previous headaches. It does not evolve from a pre-existing, episodic form of headache. For some people, the onset follows a triggering event, such as an infection, flu-like illness, surgery or stressful life event. But for more than one-third of people with this type of chronic daily headache, there is no recognized trigger.

Once it begins in this memorable fashion, new daily persistent headache occurs — as its name indicates — daily. In studies of people with this type of headache, 82 percent were able to pinpoint the exact day when their headaches began. Some people can even recall a date from 20 years ago!

Researchers believe there may be two forms of this headache — one that goes away within several months without treatment and another that persists despite aggressive treatment. The long-term form can continue for years without letup.

In most people with new daily persistent headache, the headache continues unabated throughout the day. The pain is usually moderate and may be described as throbbing, dull, achy, stabbing or burning, or as a pressure or tightness. Often the signs and symptoms are similar to those of other types of chronic daily headache, such as CDH in migraine, although people with new daily persistent headache tend to be slightly younger than people with the other types of CDH.

Because new daily persistent headache can last for years or even decades after it begins, it can be an extremely disabling condition. Even with aggressive treatment, many people with this headache don't improve.

Hemicrania continua

Hemicrania continua is a relatively rare type of chronic daily headache. The pain occurs on one side of the head and varies in intensity without ever disappearing completely. The pain is usually moderate but may include jolts of severe, "ice-pick" pain that last less than a minute. Rarely, the pain may alternate from one side of the head to the other.

At times, the flare-ups of severe pain are accompanied by one or more of the following symptoms on the same side as the pain:

• Tearing of the eye
• Redness of the eye
• Swelling or drooping of the eyelid
• Stuffy or runny nose

People with hemicrania continua may also have symptoms associated with migraine, such as nausea, vomiting, light sensitivity, noise sensitivity and aura.

Hemicrania continua may occur in either an episodic form or a chronic form. In the episodic form, periods of time — usually months — with daily headaches alternate with periods with no headaches. In the chronic form, headaches occur daily with little or no break, sometimes for years.

Medication overuse and rebound headaches

When you have a headache, it's a natural impulse to reach for the quick fix of a pain reliever. The more frequent your headaches are, the more pain medications you may find yourself taking. You may even start using pain medications to prevent an anticipated attack. Perhaps you're worried about missing work or a social event.

What many people don't realize is that overusing pain relievers may cause rebound headaches — recurrent headaches that develop as your body adapts to the medication. Too much medication may confuse your brain's ability to sense and respond to pain. When the effect of the medication wears off, your brain registers pain messages and the headache returns. You then take the medicine again, setting up a vicious cycle. Your body also may develop a tolerance to high levels of medication, so that you'll need to continue increasing the dose to achieve a pain-relieving effect.

Your body can become dependent on pain relievers without you even realizing it. If you use a pain medication for headaches more than two days a week, your episodic headache can transform into a chronic daily headache due to the overuse of this medication. And any existing form of chronic daily headache may be exacerbated by medication overuse.

What medications cause rebound headaches?

Almost any medication that's used for the immediate relief of headache symptoms can contribute to rebound headaches, including over-the-counter analgesics such as aspirin, acetaminophen (Tylenol, others) and ibuprofen (Advil, Motrin, others). Caffeine, an ingredient in many pain medications and dietary products, can also be a factor. But the medications that are most strongly linked to rebound headaches include:

Analgesic combinations. These drugs often contain a combination of caffeine, aspirin and acetaminophen and are well known for causing rebound headaches. The group includes prescription medications such as Fioricet, Fiorinal and Esgic, which also contain the sedative butalbital.

Migraine medications. Drugs developed specifically to treat migraine include the different triptan agents and ergotamine (Ergomar).

Opiates. Painkillers derived from opium or from synthetic opium compounds include combinations of codeine and acetaminophen (Tylenol With Codeine No. 3 and No. 4).

Signs and symptoms

Headaches caused by medication overuse occur almost every day and typically persist throughout the day. Each attack can vary in intensity, duration and location of pain. The headaches may be mild and punctuated by episodes of more severe pain, particularly at the beginning as the medication begins to wear off. They're often provoked by light physical or mental effort. And they may be accompanied by nausea, restlessness, anxiety, irritability, memory problems, difficulty in concentrating and depression. Your headaches may awaken you in the early hours of the morning. For people with migraine, rebound headaches may resemble severe, prolonged migraine attacks.

Who's at risk?

Anyone who has a history of migraine or tension-type headache is at risk of developing rebound headaches from the overuse of pain relievers. Interestingly, people who are not prone to headaches and who use daily pain medications to treat ailments such as arthritis don't usually get rebound headaches. This suggests that a susceptibility to one of the primary types of headaches also may predispose a person to headaches from medication overuse.

Breaking the cycle

To break the cycle of rebound headaches, you'll need to restrict how much pain medication you use. Depending on what drug you've been taking, you may be advised to temporarily stop using pain medications altogether or to reduce your medication use until you're taking the drug no more than twice a week.

Kicking the habit isn't easy. When you start, you can expect the headache pain to feel worse before it feels better, probably for several days. You may experience withdrawal symptoms such as nervousness, restlessness, nausea, vomiting, insomnia, abdominal pain, and diarrhea or constipation. But the frequency and intensity of the headaches should start to lessen within a week to 10 days. With perseverence, most people can experience relief from the rebound headache cycle within two months.

You may want to undergo this process under a doctor's supervision. Various treatments are available to alleviate headache pain and the side effects associated with drug withdrawal. Preventive medications are often started at the same time that you stop or reduce taking pain relievers. Preventive drugs don't have the same potential to cause rebound headaches as the acute medications. But preventive medications will probably not be fully effective until you've eliminated the overused medications from your system. This may take three to eight weeks.

A short hospital stay may be recommended for some people who are overusing medications if they:

- Have failed to stop using the medications after outpatient treatment
- Have another significant medical or psychiatric condition, such as diabetes, depression or anxiety
- Are using high dosages of drugs with butalbital or opiates
- Are abusing substances such as tranquilizers or decongestants
- Are experiencing prolonged, unrelenting headaches with other symptoms, such as nausea and vomiting

Once the rebound headache cycle is broken, you may revert back to your previous pattern of headaches, such as the occasional migraine or tension-type headache. At that point, you can work with your doctor to set up a long-term headache management plan. Daily preventive therapy may be recommended, and specific pain-relief medications can be administered carefully during future headache attacks.

Some people continue to experience frequent headaches even after stopping the overuse of medications and implementing other forms of treatment. Pain rehabilitation may be an option for them, which involves stopping the use of all medications and seeking alternative, nondrug treatments.

Treatment

Treatment for chronic daily headache focuses on preventing headaches rather than treating the acute symptoms. Specific strategies depend on which type of headache you have and on whether medication overuse is contributing to these headaches. If you're taking pain relievers more than two days each week, the first step in treatment may be to discontinue the use of these drugs. Many people with CDH also have a mood disorder, such as depression, anxiety or bipolar disorder. Treating these conditions is an important component in the overall management of headache disorders. You may be asked to keep a headache diary to help identify headache triggers and plan your treatment.

Acute medications

People with chronic daily headache may have need for pain relief medications, such as triptans and ergotamine for migraine. However, use of these drugs should be strictly limited — to no more than two days a week — to avoid medication overuse and rebound headaches. Your doctor can recommend medications that are less likely to cause rebound headaches.

Preventive medications

A variety of preventive medications may be used to treat CDH. Which drug your doctor prescribes will depend on the type of chronic daily headache you have. Preventive drugs typically take several weeks to build up in your system and become fully effective. One of the following medications may be recommended:

Antidepressants. Tricyclic antidepressants, including amitriptyline (Elavil), nortriptyline (Aventyl, Pamelor) and doxepin (Sinequan), are the most widely used treatments for all forms of CDH except hemicrania continua. These medications can also help treat the depression, anxiety and sleep disturbances that often accompany chronic daily headache. There's evidence to suggest that other antidepressants, such as the selective serotonin reuptake inhibitor (SSRI) fluoxetine (Prozac), may be an effective treatment for some individuals.

Beta blockers. These drugs, commonly used to treat high blood pressure, are also a mainstay for treating episodic migraine. Beta blockers include atenolol (Tenormin), metoprolol (Lopressor, Toprol), nadolol (Corgard), propranolol (Inderal) and timolol (Blocadren). Sometimes, they may be prescribed in combination with antidepressants for better results.

Anti-seizures. Anticonvulsant medications are used to prevent migraine and now are being used increasingly for people with CDH. These drugs include divalproex (Depakote), gabapentin (Neurontin) and topiramate (Topamax).

Muscle relaxants. Muscle relaxants such as tizanidine (Zanaflex) sometimes have been found to be effective in managing CDH.

NSAIDs. Nonsteroidal anti-inflammatory drugs, such as naproxen (Aleve, Anaprox), ketoprofen (Orudis), mefenamic acid

Treating hemicrania continua

Hemicrania continua headaches improve dramatically in response to the nonsteroidal anti-inflammatory drug indomethacin (Indocin, others). The response usually occurs within a few days. This drug can be used daily by people with hemicrania continua without fear of rebound headaches.

Some people are able to use indomethacin for several months and then gradually stop using the drug and remain free of pain. Others require long-term treatment with the medication. Because indomethacin can cause stomach ulcers, doctors often prescribe a treatment plan that includes a medication that protects the lining of the stomach. Other medications that can occasionally be helpful are ibuprofen (Advil, Motrin, others), piroxicam (Feldene), and the COX-2 inhibitors celecoxib (Celebrex), rofecoxib (Vioxx) and valdecoxib (Bextra).

(Ponstel) and fenoprofen (Nalfon), may be effective, especially when undergoing withdrawal from other pain relievers.

COX-2 inhibitors. Although these medications are similar to NSAIDs, they work in a different manner and with fewer side effects. Medications such as celecoxib (Celebrex), rofecoxib (Vioxx) and valdecoxib (Bextra) are most useful in people with CDH when combined with other preventive medications. They're typically prescribed for one or two months when someone is withdrawing from pain relief medications, to help decrease the frequency and severity of rebound headaches.

Others. Methysergide (Sansert) has proven to be effective in preventing migraine, but the drug is no longer available in the United States. Botulinum toxin type A (Botox) is being investigated as a possible preventive treatment for CDH.

Unfortunately, some people with chronic daily headaches don't get better, even after stopping medication overuse. Their headaches remain resistant even to preventive medications. Some of these people return to using acute medications more than two days a week. Researchers are exploring why some CDH doesn't improve with treatment and how the condition can be treated more effectively.

Nonmedication therapy

Many nonmedication strategies can help in dealing with chronic daily headache. These strategies are an essential part of any headache management plan. Nonmedication therapies are discussed in greater detail in Chapter 7. They include:

- Avoidance of known headache triggers
- No smoking
- Regular sleeping, eating and exercise habits
- Relaxation training
- Cognitive therapy
- Good posture
- Physical therapy

Stopping smoking is particularly important for people with chronic daily headache with migraine and chronic tension-type headache. Smoking can trigger both of these types of headaches. Higher levels of nicotine are also associated with increased anxiety and depression.

Sleep disorders and chronic daily headache

Headaches and sleep disorders often go hand in hand — severe headaches can disrupt your sleep, and sleep disorders can contribute to headaches. Research shows an association between headaches and sleep apnea, a condition in which a sleeper's normal breathing is repeatedly obstructed. This causes the sleeper to wake briefly and gasp for breath. Some people with CDH who also have sleep apnea find that their headaches improve when their sleep disorder is treated.

A preliminary study also found that people with chronic daily headache are almost three times more likely to be habitual snorers than people who get headaches only once in a while. Since snoring is a common symptom of sleep apnea, the findings suggest that CDH may be related to the sleep disorder in some people. More research needs to be done to support these findings and to determine what treatments might be effective.

Chapter 10

Cluster headache and related headaches

Cluster headache has the dubious distinction of being one of the most painful types of headache. Thankfully, cluster headaches are rare, affecting less than 1 percent of the U.S. population. They're more common in men, although recent studies suggest that rates of cluster headache are higher in women than previously thought. Cluster headache can affect people at any age but are most common between adolescence and middle age.

Although cluster headache attacks are extremely painful, they're not life-threatening. With proper care, most people cope well with the condition. Several treatments are currently available that can help make the attacks shorter and less severe. Preventive medications work well to reduce the number of headaches. And new treatment options are being investigated.

Cluster periods and remissions

A cluster headache is distinctive in ways other than the severity of the pain. A striking feature of cluster headache is that the attacks occur in cyclical patterns, or "clusters" — which gives the condition its name. Bouts of frequent attacks, in what's known as cluster periods, may last from weeks to months, followed by remission periods when the headache attacks stop completely. Although the pattern varies from one person to another, most people have one or two cluster periods a year. During remission, no headaches occur for months, and sometimes even years.

A cluster period generally lasts from two to 12 weeks. Chronic cluster periods may continue for more than a year. The starting date and the duration of each cluster period often are amazingly consistent from period to period. For many people, cluster periods occur seasonally, such as every spring or every fall. It's common for clusters to begin soon after one of the solstices — the longest and shortest days of the year. Over time, cluster periods may become more frequent, less predictable and longer lasting.

During a cluster period, headaches typically occur every day, sometimes several times a day. A single attack lasts 45 to 90 minutes on average. The attacks happen often at the same time within each 24-hour day. Nighttime attacks are more frequent than daytime attacks, often occurring 90 minutes to three hours after you fall asleep. The most common times for attacks are between 1 a.m. to 2 a.m., between 1 p.m. to 3 p.m., and around 9 p.m.

Types

Based on the length of the cluster periods and the remission periods, the International Headache Society has classified cluster headache into two types: episodic and chronic.

Episodic. In this form, cluster headache occurs daily for one week to one year, followed by a pain-free remission period lasting weeks to years before another cluster period develops.

Chronic. In this form, cluster headache occurs daily for more than a year with no remission or with pain-free periods lasting less than two weeks.

About 10 percent to 15 percent of people with cluster headache have the chronic type. Chronic cluster headache may develop after a period of episodic attacks, or it may develop spontaneously, without a prior history of headaches. Some people experience alternating episodic and chronic phases.

Cluster headache is one of a group of headaches called trigemi-nal autonomic cephalalgias (TACs). *Cephalalgia* (sef-uh-LAL-juh) is simply another way to say "headache" (it stems from the Greek word *kephalalgia*, meaning "head pain"). TACs can occur daily, like the chronic daily headaches discussed in Chapter 9, but they form a separate category because all feature a response of the autonomic nervous system (explained on page 112). TACs other than cluster headache are discussed later in this chapter.

Signs and symptoms

Whether you have the episodic form or the chronic form of cluster headache, the pain is the same — terrible! A cluster headache strikes quickly, usually without warning. Within minutes, excruciat-ing pain develops, generally lasting between 45 and 90 minutes, although rarely some headaches last as long as three hours. The pain affects one side of the head, usually centered behind or around the eye but may extend from the temple to the neck.

Pain typically develops on the same side of the head throughout a cluster period, and often the headaches remain on that side throughout a person's life. Less frequently, the pain may switch to the opposite side of the head in the next cluster period. Rarely, the pain switches sides from one attack to another.

The pain of a cluster headache is often described as sharp, pene-trating or burning. People with this condition say that the pain feels like a hot poker being stuck in the eye or that the eye is being push-ed out of its socket. Cluster headache has been termed the "suicide headache," because some people have contemplated suicide because of it.

Cluster headache can be frightening to the person affected by it and to his or her family and friends. The debilitating attacks may seem unendurable. But the pain usually ends as suddenly as it begins, with rapidly decreasing intensity. After attacks, most people are completely free from pain but exhausted. Temporary relief dur-ing a cluster period may be only a matter of hours or may last as long as a day before the next attack.

Restlessness

People with cluster headache appear restless, preferring to pace or sit and rock back and forth to soothe the attack. They may press a hand against the eye or scalp or apply ice or heat over the painful area. In contrast to migraineurs, people with cluster headache usually avoid lying down during an attack because this position seems to only increase the pain.

Most people with a cluster headache prefer to be alone. They may remain outdoors, even in freezing weather, for the duration of an attack. They may scream, bang their head against a wall or hurt themselves in some way as a distraction from the unbearable pain. Some may find relief by exercising, such as jogging in place or doing sit-ups or push-ups.

If cluster headache attacks regularly occur at night, some people try to remain awake for as long as possible to forestall the onset of a headache they know is coming. Unfortunately, doing so only speeds up the sleep cycle. The headache may occur within minutes of falling asleep because the REM phase comes more quickly in a compressed sleep cycle. In the worst cases, a vicious cycle of head pain and sleep deprivation develops. This can lead to depression and thoughts of suicide.

Teary eye and stuffed nose

Cluster headache always triggers a response from the autonomic nervous system. This system controls many vital activities without your consciously having to think about them. For example, it regulates blood pressure, heartbeat, sweating and body temperature. The most common autonomic response to a cluster headache is excessive tearing and redness of the eye on the side of the head affected by the pain (see page C4 of the Color Section). Other signs and symptoms that may accompany cluster headache include:

- Stuffy or runny nasal passage in the nostril on the affected side of the face
- Red, flushed face
- Swelling around the eye on the affected side of the face
- Reduced pupil size
- Drooping eyelid

Cluster headache triggers

Unlike migraine and tension-type headache, cluster headache generally isn't associated with triggers such as foods, hormonal changes or stress. But many people with cluster headache are heavy drinkers and cigarette smokers. Once a cluster period begins, consumption of alcohol can trigger a splitting headache within minutes. All it takes is one drink. For this reason, many people with cluster headache stay completely away from alcohol for the duration of a cluster period. Other possible triggers include the use of medications such as nitroglycerin — a drug used to treat heart disease.

The beginning of a cluster period often follows occasions when normal sleep patterns are disrupted, such as during a vacation or when starting a new job or work shift. Some people with cluster headache also have sleep apnea, a condition in which the walls of a person's throat collapse momentarily, obstructing the sleeper's breathing repeatedly during the night.

Most of the time, these signs and symptoms last only as long as the headache lasts. In some people, however, a drooping eyelid and reduced pupil size persist after long periods of attacks. Some migraine-like symptoms, including nausea, sensitivity to light and sound, and aura, may occur with a cluster headache.

Causes

Researchers point to different mechanisms to explain the major characteristics of cluster headache — the intense pain, the associated symptoms such as teary eye and nasal congestion, and the cyclical pattern of the attacks. In addition, recent studies indicate a family history of cluster headache in about 7 percent of people with this condition, meaning there may be a genetic component. This suggests that several factors may work together to produce cluster headache (and perhaps the other forms of trigeminal autonomic cephalalgias, or TACs).

Increased sensitivity of the nerve pathways for pain

The intense pain of a cluster headache is centered behind or around the eye, an area that's served by the trigeminal nerve, a major pathway for pain. Stimulation of this nerve results in abnormal reactions of the arteries that supply blood to the head. These blood vessels dilate and become painful.

Actions of the autonomic nervous system

Some symptoms of cluster headache, such as teary eye, stuffy or runny nose and droopy eyelid, involve the autonomic nervous system. The nerves that are part of this system form a pathway at the base of the brain. When the trigeminal nerve is activated, causing eye pain, autonomic nerves are also activated in what is called the trigeminal-autonomic reflex. Researchers believe that a still unidentified process involving inflammation or abnormal blood vessel activity in this region may also be involved in the headache.

Abnormal function of the hypothalamus

Cluster attacks typically occur with clock-like regularity during a 24-hour day. The cycle of cluster periods often follow the seasons of the year. These patterns suggest that the body's biological clock is involved. In humans, the biological clock is located in the hypothalamus, which lies deep in the center of the brain. Among the many functions of the hypothalamus is control of the sleep-wake cycle and other internal rhythms.

Abnormalities of the hypothalamus may explain the timing and cyclical nature of cluster headache. Studies have detected increased activity in the hypothalamus during the course of a cluster headache (see page C4 of the Color Section). This activity is not seen in people with headaches such as migraine.

Studies also indicate that people have abnormal levels of certain hormones, including melatonin and testosterone, during cluster periods. These hormonal changes are believed to be due to a problem with the hypothalamus. Other studies reveal that participants with cluster headache have a larger hypothalamus, compared with that of participants who don't have this headache. But it remains unknown what causes these abnormalities in the first place.

Other types of TAC headache

Other short-duration headaches are characterized by sharp, stabbing pain and symptoms such as teary eye and runny nose, similar to what happens during cluster headache. Like cluster headache, these headaches involve the trigeminal nerve and the autonomic nervous system, and so they're also classified as TACs (trigeminal autonomic cephalalgias).

Besides cluster headache, TACs include paroxysmal hemicrania (par-ok-SIZ-mul hem-ee-KRA-nee-uh) and short-lasting unilateral neuralgiform headache with conjunctival injection and tearing. The name of this latter headache is such an awkward mouthful that it's more commonly known by the acronym SUNCT. Another type of headache, hemicrania continua, has TAC characteristics but is classified as a chronic daily headache (see Chapter 9).

Attacks of paroxysmal hemicrania and SUNCT tend to be shorter and more frequent than cluster headache attacks. Like cluster headache, these TACs often occur during sleep and may be triggered by alcohol. Despite these similar features, it's not known if all TACs have a common underlying cause.

Paroxysmal hemicrania
Paroxysmal refers to a sudden occurrence or intensification of symptoms. True to its name, paroxysmal hemicrania occurs in frequent, intense but short-lasting attacks. The severe pain is on one side of the head, usually near the eye or at the temple. It has been described as stabbing, penetrating or throbbing. Autonomic signs and symptoms include redness of the eye, tearing, stuffy or runny nose, and swelling or drooping eyelid.

The pain typically lasts from two to 45 minutes. And most people have five or more attacks each day, with some people reporting as many as 40 attacks a day. In contrast to people with cluster headache, those with paroxysmal hemicrania can usually sit quietly or lie in their beds.

This type of headache is more common in women than in men. It may be chronic, with no remission. Or it may be episodic, with periods of frequent attacks separated by periods of remission.

Bouts of paroxysmal hemicrania usually subside in response to the nonsteroidal anti-inflammatory drug indomethacin (Indocin), when used as a preventive agent. Other NSAIDs as well as calcium channel blockers also may be effective.

SUNCT

This short-duration headache is one of the rarest forms of head pain. Most people affected by SUNCT are men. The pain occurs in brief episodes lasting from five seconds to about four minutes. Most people have five to six attacks in an hour, although some people may have as many as 30 episodes in an hour.

The pain of a SUNCT headache is usually on one side of the head, behind or around the eye. The pain is moderately severe and may be stabbing or throbbing. The most prominent autonomic feature is a reddened eye, and the eye also may water.

SUNCT is difficult to treat. Most drugs that work well for other short-duration headaches aren't useful for this type of headache, though anti-seizure medications such as lamotrigine (Lamictal) and topiramate (Topamax) may be effective for some people.

Other short-duration headaches

Short-duration headaches other than cluster headache, paroxysmal hemicrania and SUNCT are not categorized under the TAC designation. That's because they don't include a prominent response from the autonomic nervous system, such as teary eye or stuffy nose. These headaches include hypnic headache, trigeminal neuralgia and stabbing headache.

Hypnic headache is a rare condition that primarily affects older adults, usually a few hours after they go to sleep at night. These headaches are discussed in Chapter 15. Trigeminal neuralgia is characterized by brief attacks of facial pain, usually lasting only seconds. This condition is discussed in Chapter 11.

Stabbing headache is sometimes referred to as ice-pick headache because of brief, extremely sharp twinges of pain. People describe the pain as if their head is being stabbed or jabbed or as if the point of a spike is being driven into the skull. The stabs of pain occur without warning and may affect any part of the head. Stabbing headache may develop spontaneously, or it may accompany another type of headache, such as migraine or cluster headache. Suddenly changing your posture, doing physical exertion or going from darkness to light may trigger a stabbing headache.

Because the pain of stabbing headache is brief and occurs occasionally, treatment often isn't required. If pain does occur frequently or persistently, however, the headaches can be treated effectively with indomethacin (Indocin).

Treatment

Because the pain of a cluster headache comes on suddenly and may subside within a short time, over-the-counter pain relievers such as aspirin or ibuprofen aren't effective. The headache is usually gone before the drug starts working. Fortunately, other types of acute medication can provide some pain relief. Treatment of TACs is focused more on prevention, with more medication options available for you to choose from. In addition to medications, self-care strategies may help you avoid situations that trigger headaches.

The goal of these treatment strategies is to reduce the severity and frequency of cluster attacks. Although you can find substantial relief and prevent many attacks, the cluster periods do not disappear completely. In rare cases when medication and nonmedication strategies have little effect, surgery may be recommended.

Acute medication

Acute treatment tries to stop or reduce pain after a cluster headache starts. Because the headache peaks quickly, acute medications must be fast-acting and delivered quickly, using an injection or inhaler rather than oral tablets. You must be ready to take the medication as soon as an attack starts. And you may want to teach family members about your medications so that they'll be able to help you when you have an attack.

Oxygen. Briefly inhaling 100 percent oxygen through a mask — at a rate of seven liters per minute — provides dramatic relief for about 70 percent of people who use it. Occasionally, a higher flow rate may be more effective. The effects of this safe, inexpensive procedure can be felt within 15 minutes. The major drawback of oxygen is the need to carry an oxygen cylinder and regulator with you, which can make the treatment inconvenient and inaccessible at times. Although small, portable units are available, some people still find them impractical. Sometimes, oxygen may only delay rather than stop the attack, and pain may return.

Sumatriptan. The injectable form of sumatriptan (Imitrex), which is commonly used to treat migraine, is also an effective acute treatment for cluster headache. Some people may benefit from using sumatriptan in nasal spray form, but more studies are needed to determine the effectiveness of this approach. Sumatriptan is not recommended for people with uncontrolled high blood pressure or ischemic heart disease.

Another triptan medication, zolmitriptan (Zomig), can be taken orally for relief of cluster headache. Although oral zolmitriptan isn't as effective as injectable sumatriptan, it may be an option for people who can't tolerate other forms of acute treatment. Researchers are also investigating the use of the nasal spray form of zolmitriptan for cluster headache.

Dihydroergotamine. This ergot derivative is available in injectable and inhaler forms. Dihydroergotamine (D.H.E. 45, Migranal) is an effective pain reliever for some people with cluster headache. When administered intravenously, the drug requires you to go to a hospital or doctor's office to have an intravenous (IV) line placed. The inhaler form of the drug works more slowly. The dosage must be limited to avoid side effects, especially nausea.

Local anesthetics. The numbing effect of local anesthetics, such as lidocaine (Xylocaine), may be effective against cluster headache pain when used in the form of nasal drops.

Preventive medications

A preventive strategy is crucial for managing cluster headache because trying to treat it only with acute drugs can seem hopeless. Prevention can help reduce the frequency and severity of the attacks and the risk of rebound headaches. Preventive medications can also increase the effectiveness of acute medication.

Preventive medications for cluster headache are generally used for either a short-term (transitional) or long-term (maintenance) strategy. The short-term medications work quickly but may have undesirable side effects. Long-term medications take effect more slowly but can be used safely throughout the cluster period.

Whenever a cluster period starts, you'll start taking a long-term medication, many times accompanied by a short-term medication. After a couple of weeks, you'll discontinue use of the short-term medication but continue with the long-term drug.

Short-term prevention. Short-term medications are used to prevent headache attacks during the period of time it takes for one of the long-term drugs to become effective. The main short-term preventive medications are corticosteroids and ergotamine. A nerve block may also be effective, particularly for some people who cannot tolerate the other medications.

Corticosteroids. Inflammation-suppressing drugs called corticosteroids, such as prednisone (Deltasone, Sterapred, others) and dexamethasone (Decadron), are fast-acting preventive medications. They may be prescribed if your cluster headache condition has only recently started or if you have a pattern of brief cluster periods and long remissions. While corticosteroids are an excellent treatment for several days, serious side effects make them inappropriate for long-term use.

Ergotamine. Ergotamine (Ergomar), available as a sublingual tablet or rectal suppository, can be taken before bed to prevent nighttime attacks. Ergot medications are effective for short periods but shouldn't be used for more than two to three weeks.

Nerve block. Injecting an anesthetic (numbing agent) into the fibers around the occipital nerve, located at the back of the head, can prevent pain messages from traveling along that nerve pathway. The occipital nerve converges with the trigeminal nerve, which connects to all the pain-sensitive structures in the skull. An occipital nerve block can be useful for temporary relief until long-term preventive medications take effect.

Long-term prevention. Long-term medications are taken during the entire cluster period. About 10 percent of people with chronic cluster headache don't respond well to the use of one long-term

Self-care for cluster headache

The following measures may help you avoid a cluster attack.

Stick to a regular sleep schedule. Cluster periods often begin when there are changes in your normal sleep schedule. And during a cluster period, stay with your usual routine.

Avoid afternoon naps. Once a cluster period has started, taking an afternoon nap brings on a headache for many people.

Avoid alcohol. Alcohol, including beer and wine, almost always triggers a headache during a cluster period. This can happen quickly, even before you finish the first drink.

Limit exposure to volatile substances. Prolonged exposure to substances such as solvents, gasoline and oil-based paints may trigger an attack.

Be cautious in high altitudes. During a cluster period, the reduced oxygen at altitudes over 5,000 feet may trigger a headache. There may be drug interactions between your medications for cluster headache and medications used for mountain sickness such as acetazolamide (Dazamide, Diamox, others).

Avoid tobacco products. Nicotine may trigger a headache during a cluster period. If you're prone to cluster headache, it's best to stop smoking and avoid other tobacco products.

Avoid glare and bright lights. For some people, excessive glare and bright lights can bring on a headache.

medication. In this situation, your doctor may recommend that you take two or more long-term medications simultaneously.

Calcium channel blockers. The calcium channel blocking agent verapamil (Calan, Covera, Isoptin) is often the first choice for preventing cluster headache, although the way verapamil works with cluster headache is not well understood. The medication may be used from the start of a cluster period until three to four weeks after the last headache. Then its use is gradually tapered and discontinued under your doctor's direction. Occasionally longer-term use is needed to manage chronic headache. Constipation is a common side effect of this medication, as well as dizziness, nausea, fatigue, swelling of the ankles and low blood pressure.

Lithium carbonate. Lithium (Lithobid), which is used to treat bipolar disorder, is also effective in preventing chronic cluster headache. Side effects include tremor, increased thirst, diarrhea and drowsiness. Your doctor can adjust the dosage to minimize side effects. While you're taking this medication, your blood will be drawn at regular intervals to check for the development of more serious side effects, such as liver or kidney damage.

Other medications. Promising preventive medications for cluster headache include the hormone melatonin, capsaicin (Zostrix) — a cream that affects nerves near the skin — and anti-seizure medications such as divalproex (Depakote), gabapentin (Neurontin) and topiramate (Topamax). Injections of botulinum toxin type A (Botox), a wrinkle-smoothing drug, may provide relief for some people with cluster headache who don't respond to conventional medication. More studies are needed to evaluate the effectiveness of all these treatments for cluster headache.

Surgery

Rarely, surgery is recommended for people with chronic cluster headache who don't respond well to aggressive treatment or who can't tolerate the medications or their side effects. Candidates for surgery must have headaches only on one side of the head — because the surgery can be performed only once. People with headaches that alternate sides of the head risk the chance that the procedure will be unsuccessful.

Several types of surgery have been used to treat cluster headache. These procedures attempt to damage the nerve pathways thought to be responsible for pain. However, residual muscle weakness in your jaw or sensory loss in certain areas of your face and head may occur as a result. The most common procedures are directed at the trigeminal nerve.

Using a conventional invasive procedure, the surgeon cuts part of the trigeminal nerve with a scalpel or uses small burns to destroy part of the nerve. This form of surgery provides relief for about 75 percent of people with chronic cluster headache.

In a procedure called radiosurgery, a focused beam of radiation is used to destroy part of the trigeminal nerve. Radiosurgery is a noninvasive procedure with fewer side effects than conventional surgery, but the effectiveness, safety and permanency of the results aren't well established.

Promising approaches

As investigators learn more about the causes of cluster headache, they're able to develop more selective treatments for the condition. A recent development that shows promise is the use of a device to stimulate the occipital nerve, which influences the trigeminal nerve. To treat people with frequent cluster headaches, researchers are testing a stimulator — a pacemaker-sized device that sends impulses via electrodes — that is implanted over the occipital nerve. With the stimulator in place, the recipient's attacks may subside and he or she can remain pain free for months.

Similar research is under way using an implanted stimulator in the hypothalamus, the area of the brain associated with the timing of cluster periods. Stimulation of the hypothalamus in an individual with severe, chronic cluster headache produced complete and long-term pain relief with no significant side effects.

In addition, new medications are being studied for use in treating and preventing cluster headache. In all, researchers are hopeful that soon they'll have more effective tools to combat this particularly devastating type of headache.

Chapter 11

Trigeminal neuralgia and other neuralgias

Imagine having a lightning-quick jab of pain shoot along the side of your face unexpectedly as you talk to a friend. Unfortunately, for the thousands of people who have trigeminal neuralgia (tri-JEM-ih-nul noo-RAL-juh), they don't have to imagine this scenario. These excruciatingly painful attacks are all too familiar.

Neuralgia is pain that follows the path of a specific nerve, possibly as a result of irritation or damage, but many times the cause is unknown. The International Headache Society includes several forms of neuralgia that affect the facial area in its headache classification system. Trigeminal neuralgia refers to pain in the facial areas served by the fifth cranial (trigeminal) nerve. The condition also is known as tic douloureux (TIK doo-loo-ROO), meaning "painful tic," because people who have this condition often grimace when the pain strikes — as if they have a facial tic.

The initial attacks of trigeminal neuralgia may be mild. However, the condition can quickly progress, causing more frequent and severe pain. Fully developed, trigeminal neuralgia is one of the most painful conditions that a person can experience. The attacks may be spontaneous, but they may also start from mild stimulation of your face, including brushing your teeth or putting on makeup. The pain tends to concentrate in a small area of your face or mouth, but after frequent attacks it may expand to a wider area.

Although trigeminal neuralgia can be extremely painful, the condition usually can be controlled with medication and, possibly, surgical procedures. See your doctor if you experience any of the signs and symptoms of trigeminal neuralgia described below.

Signs and symptoms

An attack of trigeminal neuralgia may last anywhere from a few seconds to about a minute. Some people feel occasional, mild twinges of pain, while others have frequent, severe pain that feels like an electric shock. Some people with initially mild attacks may develop more severe episodes of jolting, piercing pain.

People who have experienced severe forms of trigeminal neuralgia describe the pain as lightning-like, shooting, jabbing, sharp and electric. Trigeminal neuralgia most often affects one side of the face — the right side a bit more commonly than the left. When it does affect both sides, the pain doesn't occur at the same time on both sides. While the pain can occur in the upper face, it usually affects the area of the nose, mouth, lips and cheeks.

The condition tends to come and go. Attacks may occur several times a day, or they may be more frequent, occurring one after

---

Triggers of trigeminal neuralgia pain

Many normal, everyday activities may trigger trigeminal neuralgia. It can be anything involving mild stimulation of your face. The activity may be no more than the motion of your jaw opening and closing or the application of light pressure on the trigger area. Here are some commonly identified triggers:

- Eating
- Drinking
- Talking
- Smiling
- Brushing your teeth
- Putting on makeup

- Shaving
- Stroking your face
- Encountering a slight breeze
- Walking into an air-conditioned room

another for hours or days at a time. Then a prolonged period of time with no painful attacks may follow. More than 50 percent of people with trigeminal neuralgia will have a remission period of at least six months during their lifetimes.

Trigeminal neuralgia affects women slightly more than it affects men. It's also experienced primarily by older adults. In 90 percent of cases, the condition begins after the age of 40.

Causes

The pain of trigeminal neuralgia results from a disturbance in the trigeminal nerve. From its origin deep inside your brain, this large nerve divides into three branches, which carry physical sensations from your face to your brain:

- The first branch transmits sensations from your eye, upper eyelid and forehead.
- The second branch transmits sensations from your lower eyelid, cheek, nostril, upper lip and upper gum.
- The third branch transmits sensations from the jaw, lower lip and lower gum, and innervates or stimulates the muscles you use for chewing.

You may feel pain in an area served by one branch of the trigeminal nerve or the pain may spread across a wider area served by two or all three branches. In many cases, the cause of facial pain is a blood vessel coming in contact with and irritating the trigeminal nerve (see page C5 of the Color Section). Less common causes include tumors and multiple sclerosis, although in some cases, there's no identifiable cause.

Diagnosis

Some people mistake the pain of trigeminal neuralgia for a toothache. That's understandable in instances where the pain seems to stem from your gums. It's also possible to associate the pain of trigeminal neuralgia with the onset of a headache. Nevertheless, if you experience facial pain, particularly if the pain is severe or it doesn't go away with the use of over-the-counter medication, consider seeing your doctor.

Because there are no tests to detect trigeminal neuralgia, diagnosing the disorder starts by ruling out other potential problems. Your doctor will ask about your medical history and have you describe the pain. How severe is it? How long does it last? What part of your face does it affect? And what seems to trigger the episodes? Your doctor will examine your face to try to determine exactly where the pain is occurring and — if it appears you have trigeminal neuralgia — which branch or branches of the trigeminal nerve may be affected.

Following the interview and physical examination, your doctor may be able to exclude other possible conditions that could be causing the pain. To be sure, he or she also may resort to magnetic resonance imaging (MRI) of your head. MRI is performed to check for conditions such as tumors or multiple sclerosis. MRI may occasionally help to determine whether a blood vessel is compressing your trigeminal nerve. If your doctor is able to diagnose your condition as trigeminal neuralgia, he or she can recommend a treatment that's best suited to help you manage the pain.

Treatment

Doctors usually can help you manage trigeminal neuralgia effectively with either medications or surgery. The goal of this treatment is to decrease the frequency of attacks and severity of pain with the fewest side effects.

Medications

The initial treatment for trigeminal neuralgia starts with medications. A number of drug options are available that may effectively lessen or block the pain signals being sent along the nerve pathway. If you stop responding to a particular medication or experience too many side effects from use, it's possibile that you can switch to another medication.

Carbamazepine. The anti-seizure drug carbamazepine (Carbatrol, Tegretol) is the most effective treatment for trigeminal neuralgia. In its early stages, about 75 percent of those individuals who take carbamazepine respond well to the initial treatment. The effectiveness of carbamazepine can decrease over time. Side effects include dizziness, double vision, sleepiness and nausea.

Phenytoin. Phenytoin (Dilantin, Phenytek), another anti-seizure drug, produces positive results about 60 percent of the time in people with trigeminal neuralgia. Its effectiveness may increase when used in combination with carbamazepine or baclofen. Side effects include lack of coordination, swollen gums and drowsiness.

Baclofen. Baclofen (Lioresal) is a muscle relaxant. Its effectiveness may increase when used in combination with carbamazepine or phenytoin. Side effects include confusion, mental depression and drowsiness.

Oxcarbazepine and gabapentin. Both oxcarbazepine (Trileptal) and gabapentin (Neurontin) are anti-seizure medications. Side effects may include dizziness, blurred vision and fatigue.

If any of these medications are not effective or you experience side effects, other medications may be used including clonazepam (Klonopin), divalproex (Depakote), lamotrigine (Lamictal) and topiramate (Topamax).

Over time, some people with trigeminal neuralgia stop responding to medications they've had success with or experience unacceptable side effects. For these people, surgery — sometimes combined with medications — may be an option.

Surgical procedures

For about one-third to one half of individuals who have trigeminal neuralgia, the condition will progress to a point where surgery may be considered. The procedure generally is performed by a neurosurgeon. Because most surgical procedures intend to damage the part of the trigeminal nerve that's causing pain, a side effect of these procedures is facial numbness of varying degrees. The surgical procedures include:

Alcohol injection. Injections of alcohol under the skin into a branch of the trigeminal nerve may offer temporary pain relief by numbing the area for weeks or months. Because the pain relief isn't permanent, you may need repeated injections.

Glycerol injection. In this procedure, called glycerol rhizotomy, the surgeon inserts a needle into the trigeminal cistern, a sac of fluid surrounding the trigeminal nerve. Using X-ray images to make sure that the needle is in the proper location, the doctor injects a small amount of sterile glycerol. Within three to four hours, the glycerol will have damaged the nerve and blocked pain signals.

Glycerol injection relieves pain initially in more than 80 percent of people who undergo this procedure. However, about 60 percent of those people will have a recurrence of pain, and many experience some facial numbness or tingling.

Balloon compression. In a procedure called percutaneous balloon compression, the surgeon inserts a hollow needle through the skin and into an opening in your skull. Then, a thin, flexible tube (catheter) with a balloon on the end is threaded through the needle. The balloon is inflated with enough pressure to damage the trigeminal nerve and block pain signals.

Balloon compression successfully controls pain in more than 80 percent of individuals who undergo this procedure. Up to half of these people experience a recurrence of pain. Many experience facial numbness of varying degrees, and more than half experience some damage to the motor portion of the trigeminal nerve, resulting in temporary or permanent weakness of the jaw muscles.

Electric current. A procedure called percutaneous radiofrequency thermocoagulation selectively destroys nerve fibers associated with facial pain. In a manner similar to what occurs in balloon compression, the surgeon inserts a hollow needle through your skin and into an opening in your skull. Once in place, an electrode is threaded through the needle until it rests against the trigeminal nerve root. Then an electric current is applied through the tip of the electrode for several seconds, damaging the nerve fibers.

The application of electric current controls pain in about 90 percent of people who undergo the procedure. There may be a recurrence of pain, but the application can be repeated if necessary. A common side effect of this treatment is facial numbness. The chewing muscles are sometimes weakened as well.

Microvascular decompression. Microvascular decompression doesn't damage any part of the trigeminal nerve. Instead, the procedure relocates or removes a blood vessel that may be in contact with the nerve. During the procedure, the surgeon makes an incision behind one ear at the location of a small hole in your skull. This allows part of your brain to be lifted to expose the trigeminal nerve. The surgeon repositions the blood vessel and inserts a pad to keep it separate from the nerve.

The procedure can eliminate or reduce pain about 90 percent of the time. It also provides the longest-lasting pain relief. However, pain may recur in up to 25 percent of those treated with microvascular decompression. If pain recurs, the procedure may be repeated, or a different treatment may be recommended. Microvascular decompression also carries certain risks. Although they are small, the risks include decreased hearing, facial weakness, double vision, stroke or even death. The risk of facial numbness is much less with microvascular decompression than with the procedures that intentionally damage the trigeminal nerve.

Severing the nerve. During surgery, if no blood vessel is found in contact with the trigeminal nerve, the surgeon may partially sever the trigeminal nerve to help relieve pain.

Stereotactic radiosurgery. This procedure, also known as gamma-knife radiosurgery, uses a special machine to deliver doses of high-intensity radiation to the root of the trigeminal nerve. The procedure is successful in eliminating pain about 60 percent of the time. Stereotactic radiosurgery is painless and typically is done without anesthesia. It may cause facial numbness. Because it's relatively new, the long-term outcomes still are not known.

Other neuralgias

Trigeminal neuralgia, which affects the fifth cranial nerve, is a well-known type of neuralgia. However, facial pain may develop at other locations of the face and head. Both glossopharyngeal neuralgia and postherpetic neuralgia generally affect individuals over age 40. Similar to trigeminal neuralgia, a variety of drugs, including anti-seizure medications such as carbamazepine and phenytoin, are used in treatment. Surgical procedures such as microvascular decompression and severing the nerve also may be used.

Glossopharyngeal neuralgia

Glossopharyngeal (glos-o-fuh-RIN-je-ul) neuralgia is a disturbance of the glossopharyngeal nerve, one of the cranial nerves located below the trigeminal nerve. It's characterized by brief, severe pains in your throat, tonsils, tongue and ear. The pain is usually triggered by swallowing, chewing, speaking, laughing or coughing.

Postherpetic neuralgia

Postherpetic (post-her-PET-ik) neuralgia is a common complication of shingles, which occurs when the virus that causes chickenpox is reactivated inside your nerve cells. Shingles usually heals within a month, but nerve and skin pain may last in the affected areas long after the rash and blisters heal. The pain that remains is postherpetic neuralgia.

Postherpetic neuralgia can affect any part of your body. The most common locations in the head affected by postherpetic neuralgia are the forehead and an eye on one side of the face.

Be proactive — don't wait for treatment

The searing bursts of pain of a cranial neuralgia can be incapacitating. Even if the attack lasts only for a few seconds, its effects can completely disrupt your day. The attacks come and go variably, but the time between them may grow shorter as you get older. So even if the condition seems bearable to you at the moment, plan to consult your doctor about the pain. Symptoms normally improve and stay manageable with treatment.

Chapter 12

Secondary types of headache

A headache is not always just a headache. Sometimes, head pain is a symptom of another disease, perhaps one that you may not even be aware of. Headaches that are a result of an underlying condition are called secondary headaches.

Indeed, head pain often is one of the first signs of something wrong in your body. In some cases, the problem may be nothing more than an upper respiratory infection, too much physical exertion or caffeine withdrawal. More serious headaches can result from a brain tumor or an aneurysm that forms at a weakened blood vessel wall. There are many causes of secondary headache, including sinusitis, head trauma and metabolic disorders.

Secondary headaches can mimic the steady ache of tension-type headache or the painful throb of migraine. On other occasions, they develop quite differently from a primary headache — striking with no warning or getting progressively worse over time. Secondary headaches also commonly occur along with symptoms such as fever, stiff neck, dizziness, mental confusion and seizures.

The good news is that secondary headaches are relatively rare, accounting for less than 10 percent of all headaches. Still, it's important to recognize the warning signs for these headaches and receive the proper treatment for them. Some of the most frequent causes of secondary headaches are described in this chapter.

Trauma

Headaches are one of the most common signs of injury to the head, neck or brain caused by falls, impacts during sports or on-the-job activities, auto accidents or physical assaults.

Acute headaches can begin at any time within two weeks of the trauma and last for months. The chronic form can last for two years or more. It's not clear why some headaches are slow to begin and why others last so long following an injury. The severity of the trauma seems to have little to do with it. Even mild concussions can result in painful, long-lasting headaches.

Headaches due to trauma frequently produce the band of pressure associated with tension-type headache. Less often, these headaches resemble migraine, with throbbing pain, nausea and sensitivity to light and sound. Other symptoms may include dizziness, blurred vision, insomnia, mental confusion and irritability.

If you notice any of these symptoms following a head trauma, see your doctor immediately. Sudden or severe symptoms can indicate a problem that requires emergency treatment. If no underlying

---

When a headache spells trouble

Most headaches are not cause for alarm. But if you develop headaches that are very different from ones you've had in the past, an underlying medical condition could be to blame. Seek medical care immediately if you exhibit one or more of these warning signs:

- Abrupt, severe headache, often like a thunderclap
- Headache with other signs and symptoms such as fever, stiff neck, rash, mental confusion, seizures, double vision, weakness, numbness or speaking difficulties
- Headache that you'd classify as the worst you've ever had
- Headache after a head injury, especially if it gets worse
- Headache caused by coughing, exertion, straining or a sudden movement
- A new headache pattern or a pattern that progressively gets more severe after age 50

problems are found, pain relievers such as acetaminophen (Tylenol, others) and ibuprofen (Advil, Motrin, others) may offer adequate relief. If your headache is migraine-like, medications developed specifically for migraine may be appropriate.

Nonvascular intracranial disorders

A new type of headache or the worsening of a pre-existing headache may signal a nonvascular intracranial disorder. This may be any condition that causes increased pressure within your skull (intracranial) but is unrelated to a problem with the blood vessels that supply the brain (nonvascular). Normal pressure may be altered by the abnormal growth of brain cells, an injury that causes swelling or a trauma that causes a buildup of blood. A change in the volume of cerebrospinal fluid — a clear liquid that surrounds and protects your brain and spinal cord — also can increase pressure inside your skull. Often, the conditions that produce these headaches require immediate medical treatment.

Brain tumor

A brain tumor is an abnormal mass of cells growing in the brain. Some tumors are benign, or relatively nonthreatening, while others are malignant, or more aggressive. Sometimes, a malignant tumor results from cancer that has started elsewhere in the body — such as the breast or lung — and has spread to the brain.

Although brain tumors can occur at any age, they're most common in children ages 3 to 12 and adults ages 40 to 70. A headache is a common, early symptom. The pain from these headaches may vary, depending on where the tumor is located (see page C7 of the Color Section). Sometimes, the condition may start as a morning headache. Over weeks or months, however, the pain typically becomes continuous and more severe.

Treatment for a brain tumor will depend on the type, size and location of the tumor as well as your age and overall health. However, surgery is the mainstay treatment. With malignant tumors, radiation and chemotherapy also may be used.

Hydrocephalus

Blockage of cerebrospinal fluid in and around the brain can lead to an emergency complication known as hydrocephalus (hi-dro-SEF-uh-lus). Common signs and symptoms of the condition include headache, nausea, blurred or double vision, problems with balance, and sluggishness. To relieve the pressure of fluid buildup and to reduce the risk of brain injury, this fluid must be drained.

Subdural hematoma

Head trauma can cause veins along the brain's surface to stretch and tear. Tearing allows blood to collect beneath the outer covering of the brain (the dura mater). This condition is known as subdural hematoma (see page C6 of the Color Section). Occasionally, the condition can occur without trauma in older adults.

Signs and symptoms include loss of consciousness, headache, weakness or numbness, slurred speech or the inability to speak, nausea and vomiting, and lethargy. If large, a subdural hematoma is an urgent condition that may cause brain damage.

Idiopathic intracranial hypertension

Although this form of hypertension increases intracranial pressure, no evidence of a tumor, infection, blood clot or blockage of spinal fluid exists (*idiopathic* means "of unknown cause"). This condition, also called pseudotumor cerebri, most often affects young, obese women. Signs and symptoms include headache, nausea and vomiting, and swelling of the optic nerve. The headache can occur daily and cause pulsating pain that gradually increases in intensity. Coughing and other sudden movement can aggravate the pain.

A procedure known as a lumbar puncture, or spinal tap, may be done one or more times to decrease pressure and headache pain (see Chapter 3). Other recommended treatments include weight loss, fluid or salt restriction, and the use of medications such as diuretics. Surgery may also be considered to relieve the pressure.

Spontaneous intracranial hypotension

Intracranial hypotension occurs when a tear in the outer covering of the brain and spinal cord causes spinal fluid to leak. Headaches are a common symptom of the condition, usually when the head is upright. Most people can be treated with pain relievers, fluids and several days of bed rest as the leak heals on its own. If the headache persists, a procedure known as a blood patch may be performed. If an infection occurs, treatment with antibiotics may be necessary.

Vascular disorders

The abnormal function of the brain's blood vessels can cause headaches. A headache also may be a symptom of an ischemic stroke, which interrupts the blood supply to the brain. Vascular disorders associated with headache include high blood pressure, aneurysm or hemorrhage within the brain, blood leakage from artery walls, and inflammation within the arteries.

High blood pressure
This condition, also called hypertension, causes higher than normal pressure within your blood vessels. A few people with high blood pressure in its early stage experience a dull ache at the back of the head when they wake in the morning. For the most part, headaches don't occur until blood pressure has become severely elevated.

Whether or not you have headaches, you should have your blood pressure checked at least every two years. If it's high, you'll need to control it. That's because the higher the pressure or the longer it goes uncontrolled, the greater the damage it can do to your blood vessels and vital organs. Lifestyle changes and medication often can reduce pressure and relieve signs and symptoms.

Cerebral aneurysm and hemorrhage
An aneurysm occurs when a weakened blood vessel wall bulges under the pressure of circulating blood. Some cerebral aneurysms are only a few millimeters across. Others can bulge large enough to put pressure on the brain, causing such symptoms as double vision, headaches and eye pain. More often, symptoms develop when the aneurysm bursts and blood leaks into the brain and spinal fluid. This leakage is called a subarachnoid hemorrhage.

Aneurysms can rupture because of head trauma, blood vessel abnormalities or high blood pressure. A sudden, severe headache — often referred to as a thunderclap headache — typically signals a ruptured aneurysm. Other symptoms may include muscle weakness, numbness, vision problems, speech impairment, mental confusion, sluggishness and seizures. Emergency treatment is needed because a rupture can be fatal.

Carotid and vertebral dissection

Two carotid arteries, located on either side of the neck, deliver blood to the brain. Sometimes, blood leaks into the artery wall and collects there, a process known as dissection (see page C7 of the Color Section). If enough blood collects, a clot can form that blocks blood flow. Usually the first sign of the condition is a headache, sometimes with pain in the face and neck. Other symptoms include drooping eyelid, small pupil size and double vision.

Another form of dissection involves the two vertebral arteries, which circulate blood to the back of the brain. Many conditions can disrupt blood flow in these arteries, including a tear in the artery wall. Symptoms include headache, nausea, vision problems, numbness, vertigo, poor coordination and difficulty with swallowing. Both forms of dissection increase the risk for stroke.

Cranial arteritis

In cranial arteritis, also known as giant cell arteritis or temporal arteritis, inflammation damages the blood vessels carrying blood throughout your body. The condition happens most often in the arteries to the head. Common symptoms of cranial arteritis are headache, jaw pain, and blurred or double vision. This condition affects older adults almost exclusively (see Chapter 14).

Sinusitis

Each year more than 30 million Americans are affected by sinusitis, a condition in which the membranes lining the sinuses become swollen and inflamed, trapping mucus in the air-filled cavities. Unable to drain properly, the mucus becomes infected, often causing pain around the eyes and across the cheeks and forehead.

Many headaches attributed to sinus problems are actually migraine or, less commonly, tension-type headache. When sinus headaches do occur, they have characteristic signs and symptoms. Sinusitis is caused by a bacterial infection and often follows a cold or allergies that cause congestion. The headaches that result typically produce severe pain in the clogged areas of the sinus cavities and occur with fever and a thick mucus discharge that's yellow-green in color. Pain may become worse if you bend forward or lie down.

If sinusitis becomes chronic, the headaches produce a dull ache over the sinus area and may occur with thick nasal discharge and a continuous flow of mucus onto the back of the throat (postnasal drip). If you have asthma, nasal polyps, or allergies to dust, mold or pollen, you may be prone to developing chronic sinusitis. The same is true if you have an immune deficiency disease or a condition such as cystic fibrosis, which affects the way mucus moves within your respiratory system.

If antibiotics can eliminate the underlying cause of the infection, the sinus headaches should disappear as well. At the same time, over-the-counter pain relievers, decongestants and nasal sprays can help alleviate many signs and symptoms. But be careful not to overuse these products. If sinus infections continue to occur, your doctor may prescribe stronger medication.

Infection of the central nervous system

Headaches are common with any type of infection. This is particularly true with infections of the brain and spinal cord. These infections include meningitis, encephalitis and AIDS. Not all infections will produce the same type of headache.

Brain abscess

A brain abscess is a mass of immune cells, pus and other materials that result from a brain infection. Although the mass isolates the infection, it also may put pressure on delicate brain tissue. Common signs and symptoms of an abscess include headache, muscle weakness, loss of coordination or balance, and seizures. If you have a condition that compromises your immune system, such as HIV, you're at higher risk for developing an abscess.

Meningitis

Meningitis is an inflammation of the membranes and fluid surrounding the brain and spinal cord caused by a bacterial, viral or fungal infection. Bacterial meningitis often results from an infection in another part of your body that spreads to the central nervous system. Intestinal viruses are a common cause of viral meningitis, but viruses associated with disease such as mumps or herpes infection may also be sources. Fungal infections are a less common cause of meningitis, occurring in people with conditions that suppress the immune system, such as AIDS.

It's easy to mistake early signs of bacterial and viral meningitis for the flu. In mild forms of viral meningitis, a fever and headache may persist over several days, but the infection usually clears on its own within a week or two. Acute forms of bacterial meningitis strike suddenly, usually with a high fever, severe headache and vomiting. Other signs and symptoms of meningitis include confusion, drowsiness, a stiff neck and seizures. If these occur, seek medical care immediately. Some types of meningitis can be fatal or lead to brain damage. Antibiotics are used to treat bacterial forms of the condition. Mild cases of viral meningitis may be treated with bed rest, fluids and analgesics that can reduce fever and body aches.

Encephalitis

Encephalitis is an inflammation of the brain caused primarily by a viral infection. Symptoms generally are mild, but they can become severe, especially with a weakened immune system. Herpes simplex encephalitis, for example, may start as a minor illness with headache and fever, followed by more serious symptoms. Mosquito-borne disease such as the West Nile virus commonly cause epidemic varieties of encephalitis. The secondary form of encephalitis accompanies a viral infection such as chickenpox, measles (rubeola), mumps, German measles (rubella) or polio.

Many times, encephalitis goes unreported because most people infected with the disease have mild or no symptoms and the illness doesn't last long. Still, the serious form can be life-threatening. Symptoms may include severe headache, sudden fever, nausea and vomiting, confusion and disorientation, and seizures.

AIDS

AIDS is a chronic, life-threatening condition caused by the human immunodeficiency virus (HIV). By damaging the cells of your immune system, HIV interferes with your body's ability to fight viruses, bacteria and fungi that cause disease. This makes you more susceptible to infections such as meningitis. By the time HIV officially develops into AIDS, you may experience persistent headaches, unexplained fatigue, soaking night sweats, shaking chills, high fever, swollen lymph nodes and chronic diarrhea. Although there is no cure for AIDS, a number of medications have been developed to treat both HIV and opportunistic infections. Some of these medications may cause side effects such as headaches.

Metabolic disorders

Some conditions may cause headaches by affecting your metabolism — how your body carries out such functions as digesting food, eliminating waste and circulating blood. For instance, headaches that occur at night could be related to disorders that restrict airflow to the lungs and decrease the amount of oxygen supplied to the brain. Causes may include everything from a lung disease such as emphysema to a sleeping disorder known as sleep apnea. Exposure to dangerous levels of carbon monoxide, which deprives your brain cells of oxygen, can cause dull morning headaches.

Headaches can result from abnormally low levels of blood sugar, or glucose, in your body (hypoglycemia). Hypoglycemia is a possible complication of your insulin treatment for diabetes. Treatment for other diabetic complications, such as kidney failure, also may lead to headaches. Another metabolic condition associated with headaches is hypothyroidism.

Other causes

Many other factors can lead to a secondary headache. These factors include problems with your eyes or your jaw, participating in strenuous exercise, and having poor eating habits.

Vision problems
Although very rare, eyestrain can be a cause of headaches, for example, from spending too many hours in front of a television or computer screen. Eyestrain also can be a problem if you use an outdated eyeglass prescription or have uncorrected vision loss. Over-the-counter pain relievers and eye rest most likely will alleviate these headaches.

A viral infection of the oculomotor nerve, which originates deep in the brain, can produce pain in one eye and paralysis of certain eye muscles. This condition, known as an ophthalmoplegic migraine, is not considered a true migraine according to the recent revision of the International Classification of Headache Disorders.

Jaw joint disorders
The temporomandibular joint is a hinge joint on each side of your skull where your lower jawbone joins with the temporal bone. Many conditions can cause pain in this joint, including simple wear and tear, arthritic inflammation, injury, stress, and poorly fitting braces or dentures. If you regularly have a headache along with tender jaw muscles, dull aching in the jaw joint, and a clicking sound or grating sensation when opening and closing your mouth, it's advisable to see your dentist. Medications such as ibuprofen (Motrin, Advil, others) and corrective dental treatment may provide relief. Appliances such as bite plates or night guards, or surgery, may help correct misaligned jaws.

Medication side effects and substance abuse
Many common antibiotics, antihistamines, decongestants and hormones have been associated with headaches. Certain medications used to treat conditions such as asthma, cardiovascular disease, depression and cancer may also cause headaches. Excessive alcohol

consumption, alcohol withdrawal and the use of illicit drugs such as cocaine have been linked to headaches.

The substances most closely associated with headaches due to overuse are analgesics (pain relievers) — the very drugs most people use to help relieve headaches. Although many OTC analgesics reduce pain quickly, they can cause problems if overused — particularly the combination drugs containing caffeine. The headaches occur once your body adapts to high levels of medication.

Physical exertion

Prolonged physical exertion can trigger headaches, typically following activities such as weightlifting, dancing, running or swimming. The throbbing pain on both sides of the head may last from five minutes to 24 hours. Hot weather and high altitudes make these headaches more likely to occur.

Headaches can also result from sudden, intense exertion while coughing, sneezing, laughing, stooping, or straining to go to the bathroom. The headache pain is often described as bursting or explosive. It usually occurs for a few seconds or minutes on both sides of the head and at the back of the skull. Exertion during sex may induce headaches. The pain, which can build during intercourse or occur before or after orgasm, may be throbbing or stabbing and last anywhere from a few minutes to an hour.

These headaches occasionally can be the sign of a medical problem such as a brain tumor or hemorrhage. More often, they're benign and can be treated with medication.

Food and eating habits

Certain foods, food additives and eating habits are frequently listed as triggers for primary headaches such as migraine. But these factors also can cause headaches with characteristics that are distinct from migraine or tension-type headache.

Hunger. If you have chronic headache or migraine, missing a meal can trigger head pain. Yet hunger-induced headaches can strike if you're normally headache-free. They often occur if you've gone without eating for 16 hours or more. To avoid hunger-induced headaches, it's important to eat regularly throughout the day.

Caffeine withdrawal. Too much caffeine in your diet can trigger headaches. Abruptly reducing caffeine consumption, however, can result in a withdrawal headache, usually within 24 to 48 hours of your last caffeinated drink. This may happen, for example, if you drink a lot of caffeine during the week and then cut back drastically on the weekend. To avoid this cycle, try to stay at moderate levels of daily caffeine intake — about three 8-ounce cups of coffee may be considered an moderate amount of caffeine.

Monosodium glutamate. Monosodium glutamate (MSG) is a food additive commonly used to enhance the flavor of Chinese food as well as many packaged, canned and frozen-food products. This additive can cause headaches soon after it's consumed, typically within 30 minutes to one hour after eating. Some people also may experience dizziness, chest pressure and abdominal cramps. If you're sensitive to MSG, ask if it's used in food preparation before ordering meals in restaurants and check the food labels when you go shopping at the grocery store.

Ice cream headaches. Eat ice cream or drink a cold beverage too quickly and you may feel almost immediate pain in your forehead. The pain may last for several seconds or minutes. An ice cream headache is more likely to occur if you're overheated from exercise or hot weather. To avoid these headaches, try taking smaller bites and warming them in the front of your mouth before swallowing.

Play it safe

It can be worrisome to think that a serious medical problem could be the cause of your headache. Thankfully, the majority of headaches are not the result of illness. But even though secondary headaches are rare, it can be dangerous to ignore head pain or symptoms that accompany them, especially if they seem out of the ordinary. If you have concerns about a headache, play it safe and contact your doctor. If your doctor does find a problem, the sooner you know what's wrong and can begin treatment, the better

Part 4

Special issues

Chapter 13

Women and headaches

Headaches are a fact of life for many women. Studies show that more than 80 percent of women of reproductive age have headaches. Not only do women get headaches more often than men do, but they also experience more severe headache symptoms. Three times as many women as men get migraine, and tension-type headache is also more common in women.

Gender differences in headache prevalence start showing up as early as puberty. In early childhood, migraine affects boys and girls equally, but after puberty, migraine is more common among women than men. Similar changes occur with tension-type headache. These patterns have led researchers to investigate the possible role played by female reproductive hormones such as estrogen in causing headaches.

The role of hormones

Why are women more prone to headaches than men are? At least part of the answer may involve hormones. Hormones are part of the endocrine system, which is a system of specialized glands. The glands produce hormones and secrete them into the bloodstream as they're needed. These hormones act as chemical messengers that help regulate many vital processes to keep you alive and functioning. They do so by relaying messages to specific organs or tissues in the body to take certain actions.

The relationship between hormones and headaches is complex and likely to be just one of several factors that play a role in producing head pain. Other contributing factors, in women and men alike, include genetic predisposition, inflammation, muscle tension and certain brain chemicals. Nevertheless, women often notice a relationship between their headaches and the major reproductive milestones of menstruation, pregnancy and menopause — precisely those times when hormone levels are fluctuating the most.

For example, the first headaches often begin around the time of a girl's first period, and many women regularly experience headaches at the time of their menstrual cycles. The use of hormones for birth control or for treatment of menopausal symptoms often coincides with headaches. Many women with migraine find that their headaches improve when they're pregnant.

The hormones most closely linked to headache in women are estrogen and progesterone, which play key roles in regulating the menstrual cycle and pregnancy. These hormones have other functions in the body, some involving the central nervous system.

Researchers believe estrogen and progesterone may help cause headaches by affecting headache-related brain chemicals. For example, high or low levels of estrogen in the blood usually correspond to high or low levels of serotonin, a brain chemical that helps regulate pain messages. In general, higher estrogen levels correlate with improvements in headaches, while lower estrogen levels result in increased headaches.

Menstruation

Studies indicate that as many as 60 percent of women with migraine report headaches in the days just before or during menstruation. Menstruation also triggers tension-type headache in 40 percent to 60 percent of women. Headache is a common symptom of premenstrual syndrome (PMS), which is a pattern of physical and emotion changes, including fatigue and anxiety, that occurs in many women just before menstruation.

The menstrual cycle involves complex, carefully orchestrated interactions among several hormones, with various effects. Although hormonal fluctuations may help trigger headaches, it bears repeating that hormones clearly aren't the whole story, since prepubescent girls and males of all ages get migraine and tension-type headache as well. As researchers explore the biological basis of menstrual headaches, they've identified one of the most common forms, called the menstrual migraine.

Menstrual migraine

The term *menstrual migraine* refers to a general migraine condition. Specific terminology describes the timing of migraine attacks during menstruation. This timing affects how the condition is treated.

Pure menstrual migraine. Headaches occur exclusively during your menstrual periods and at no other time during the cycle. This pattern involves any attack that regularly occurs within two days before and three days after the onset of your period. About seven percent of women are affected by this condition.

Menstrually associated migraine. Headaches occur throughout your cycle but increase in frequency or intensity during the time of your menstrual period.

Premenstrual migraine. Headaches occur before your menstrual period starts, generally two to seven days earlier. These headaches may be part of a premenstrual syndrome.

Seemingly at the root of menstrual migraine is the drop in estrogen that happens just before menstruation. The falling estrogen levels produce biochemical changes that increase your body's sensitivity to pain and may contribute to the headache pattern.

Signs and symptoms. The most common time for menstrual migraine to occur ranges from two days before a menstrual period begins through the first three days of the period. Signs and symptoms are similar to those of nonmenstrual migraines (see Chapter 4 for more details). Some research suggests that menstrual migraine is more severe and less responsive to treatment than migraine at other times of the month.

Aura usually doesn't accompany migraine that strikes around the time of menstruation. Premenstrual migraine may be accompanied by other signs and symptoms of PMS, including backache, anxiety, depression, crying spells, irritability, bloating, appetite changes, lethargy or fatigue, nausea, difficulty in concentrating and breast tenderness. During menstruation, migraine may coincide with abdominal pain or cramping.

Treatment. The timing of your headaches determines the treatment of menstrual migraine — whether the headaches occur before or during your period and whether they also occur at other times of the month. Keeping a headache diary can help you and your doctor identify a pattern in the migraine attacks.

Acute treatment for migraine provides immediate relief of symptoms. Preventive treatment is often recommended for women who have three or more debilitating headaches per month or whose menstrual headaches don't respond to acute medications. By definition, menstrual migraine can affect any woman in her childbearing years. If you're not using birth control or are trying to conceive, be cautious about using migraine medications since some drugs may have harmful effects on a developing fetus.

Acute treatment. Acute treatment for menstrual migraine is similar to acute treatment for other forms of migraine. Women who have a mild form of pure menstrual migraine can use over-the-counter pain relievers, with little risk of medication overuse. Nonsteroidal anti-inflammatory drugs (NSAIDs), such as naproxen (Aleve, Naprosyn, others), ketoprofen (Orudis) and mefenamic acid (Ponstel), are considered the first line of treatment.

Preventive treatment. Short-term prevention is most effective when your menstrual cycle is regular. Women who experience premenstrual migraine or pure menstrual migraine may time when they take medications, starting a few days before menstruation and continuing for the first three days of their periods. The NSAIDs commonly used for acute treatment also serve well as preventive medications. Other drugs that may be used include ergotamine and caffeine (Cafergot, Wigraine), dihydroergotamine (D.H.E. 45, Migranal) and triptans such as naratriptan (Amerge), frovatriptan (Frova) and zolmitriptan (Zomig).

Magnesium and menstrual migraine

Taking doses of magnesium, an essential mineral, to treat migraines has received considerable attention in recent years. Women with menstrual migraine have been found to have low levels of magnesium, and this deficiency may contribute to the development of headaches. Studies indicate that the use of magnesium is effective against menstrual migraine, though the benefit is likely to be small. Side effects of magnesium may include diarrhea.

Women with menstrually associated migraine — frequent attacks throughout the menstrual cycle — may use standard preventive medication that they take continuously. The same is true if your periods are difficult to predict. If you experience menstrual migraine after taking preventive medication, your doctor may prescribe higher doses in the time before your period starts.

For women with severe menstrual migraines, other forms of treatment may be recommended. These include hormonal therapies such as estrogen, most commonly taken via skin patch, and oral contraceptives. Rarely, bromocriptine (Parlodel), tamoxifen (Nolvadex), leuprolide (Lupron, Viadur) and danazol (Danocrine) may be prescribed.

Nonmedication treatments. Effective management of menstrual migraine also may involve measures such as relaxation therapy and regular sleeping, eating and exercise routines. (See Chapter 7 for more detail.) While these efforts in themselves usually aren't sufficient to treat menstrual migraine, they can improve your quality of life and may limit the frequency of attacks.

Oral contraceptives and migraines

Oral contraceptives, which usually combine estrogen and progestin (a synthetic form of progesterone), have varying effects on migraine. Some women experience their first-ever migraine attack after starting on birth control pills. If contraceptives are taken continuously, without a pill-free week, for several months by women who already have migraine, their headaches may improve. But attacks may wors-

en for other women, or the headaches may assume different characteristics. For a majority of women, however, little changes after starting oral contraceptives, especially with the lower doses of estrogen
and progestin now found in most birth control pills.

If you have a history of migraine and need to start birth control,
talk to your doctor about the risks and benefits of various forms of
contraception. If oral contraceptives seem to trigger migraine or
make the headaches worse, discuss the problem with your doctor.
Your doctor may recommend that you take a pill containing a different formulation. Unfortunately, stopping the pill may not relieve
your headaches immediately — it still may take six months to a
year before you see an improvement. Worse, your headache attacks
may not improve at all.

Other options may be to use a monthly pill pack with fewer
placebo (inactive pill) days or to eliminate the placebo days altogether from most cycles. Women who continue to experience severe
headaches while taking oral contraceptives may need to consider a
progestin-only pill or alternative forms of birth control.

Controversy surrounds the question of whether women with
migraine who use oral contraceptives are at increased risk of stroke.
If you have migraine and are considering taking birth control pills,
your doctor can evaluate your possible risk factors of stroke and
advise you on the best and safest course of action.

Pregnancy and lactation

For a majority of women who get migraine, pregnancy brings welcome relief from their headaches. Estrogen levels rise rapidly in
early pregnancy and remain high throughout the pregnancy. About
70 percent of women with migraine, especially those with menstrual migraine, experience an improvement or complete absence of
headaches during the time they're pregnant. Tension-type headache is less likely to be affected by pregnancy, with improvement
seen in only about 30 percent of women.

Sometimes, migraine symptoms may worsen in the first trimester, but then improve in the second and third trimesters, when

the estrogen levels stabilize. During some pregnancies, migraine attacks may stay the same or worsen. Migraine also may begin during pregnancy, though this is uncommon.

Headache is a common postpartum complaint. Following delivery, 40 percent of all women and 58 percent of women with migraine develop or resume having headaches, often three to six days after giving birth. Postpartum headaches may be triggered by an abrupt decrease in estrogen levels.

Treatment

The frustrating part of having headaches during pregnancy is that your treatment options are limited. Many common headache medications have potentially harmful or unknown effects on the developing fetus. Fortunately, nonmedication therapies, such as relaxation therapy, stress management, regular meals and adequate sleep, are effective for headaches. Indeed, these strategies reduce headache in 80 percent of pregnant women.

Pregnancy planning and headaches

If you get headaches regularly and are trying to conceive, don't wait until after you're pregnant to start being careful about the medications you take. Most women don't realize they're pregnant until after they've missed a period, at which point they're already several weeks along in gestation.

Many common headache medications may have adverse effects during pregnancy, especially at the time of conception. For example, NSAIDs may prevent a fertilized egg from implanting in the uterus. Other medications aren't considered safe because of unknown or possibly harmful effects on the fetus, especially during the first three months of pregnancy.

To minimize potential problems, headache specialists recommend that women with headaches plan ahead before getting pregnant. Your doctor can help you determine specific strategies for adapting your treatment program. It's not necessary to take this action months in advance — a few weeks ahead is probably fine.

In addition, many substances that pregnant women are encouraged to avoid, including alcohol, caffeine and nicotine, are considered common headache triggers. The healthy diet recommended for pregnancy also may help with headache management.

If nonmedication treatments don't help, talk to your doctor about medications that are safe to use. Headaches that persist into the second trimester are likely to continue for the remainder of the pregnancy. If the headaches are causing you distress, it's better to seek treatment than to tolerate severe pain for fear of harming the baby. Your doctor will check for other conditions that might be causing the headaches.

Aspirin is not safe to take when you're pregnant, and NSAIDs should be avoided in the first and third trimesters. Medications designed specifically for migraine, such as triptans, are not proved to be safe for use during pregnancy.

For women who have severe headaches, acetaminophen (Tylenol, others) can be used for acute pain relief during pregnancy. Other medications that may be taken are certain opiates, such as meperidine (Demerol) and codeine, and antiemetics, which are used to control nausea. Avoid overuse of these medications.

Unfortunately, the most effective medications for preventing headaches carry some risk for pregnant women. Preventive medications that are safe to use during pregnancy include selective serotonin reuptake inhibitor (SSRI) antidepressants and bupropion (Wellbutrin, Zyban). Gabapentin (Neurontin) can be used while attempting to conceive and during early pregnancy, but it should be discontinued in later pregnancy.

Lactation

Women with migraine may continue to see the same improvement in their headaches while breast-feeding as when they were pregnant. Lactation stabilizes estrogen levels and also increases the levels of other hormones that help reduce sensitivity to pain.

Women who are breast-feeding should continue to be cautious about their headache medications. Your doctor can advise you about which medications to avoid during lactation. You'll be pleased to learn that you have more options for pain relief than you did during pregnancy. That's because drug levels in breast milk are a small fraction of the drug levels that might be found in the mother's blood. Acetaminophen and caffeine are safe during breast-feeding, as are opiates and NSAIDs. Women who are breast-feeding can use injectable sumatriptan if they use a pump and discard the milk that's discharged for four hours after the injection.

Menopause

Menopause, which generally occurs between the ages of 45 and 55, is the final reproductive milestone in a woman's life. Menopause is the transition from a time when you can bear children to a time when you no longer menstruate and can no longer become pregnant. For many women, this process may continue for several months or several years as their ovaries gradually stop producing estrogen and progesterone. During the transition periods become irregular and levels of estrogen fluctuate tremendously.

Menopause, like other reproductive events, often results in changing headache patterns. Some women experience an initial worsening of headaches. This is especially true for women who've had menstrual migraine or PMS. For many other women, the headaches improve. But getting older often lessens headaches for many people — both female and male.

According to studies, more than two-thirds of women with migraine experienced an improvement in headaches after menopause. Unfortunately, these same studies indicate that migraine remained unchanged for 24 percent and worsened for other women. And a small number of women experienced their first migraines during menopause. For women whose headaches persist after menopause, pain can be treated with standard acute and preventive medications and nonmedication therapies.

Approximately two-thirds of women with migraine who underwent surgical menopause (removal of the ovaries and uterus) reported that their headaches worsened. This difference may have to do with age because women having surgical menopause generally are younger than those going through natural menopause.

Compared with migraine, tension-type headache does not improve as much when menopause comes. Among women experiencing natural menopause, tension-type headache improved in 27 percent and worsened in 60 percent.

Hormone therapy during menopause

Use of estrogen and progestin to help ease menopausal symptoms such as hot flashes and vaginal dryness is known as hormone therapy (HT), also known as hormone replacement therapy. Hormone therapy is a complex issue, which has become further complicated by findings from the Women's Health Initiative that raised serious concerns about the long-term use of Prempro, a combined estrogen and progestin pill. Short-term use of HT still may be appropriate for menopausal symptoms and seems to carry little risk. Nevertheless, the decision to use these medications can be made only after carefully discussing risks and benefits with your doctor.

About as many women using HT report an improvement in their headaches as those who report a worsening of their headaches. The effect of HT on headaches seems to depend in part on the dose and the method of administration. In general, the lowest possible dose of estrogen should be used to minimize headaches. Using an estrogen skin patch, which provides a low, steady supply, is least likely to aggravate headaches.

Every woman is unique

Fluctuating hormone levels may influence headache patterns for some women but not others as they go through menstruation, pregnancy and menopause. This supports the theory that headache pain results from a complex interplay of factors — some internal, others external. All these factors interact in different ways in different individuals, making every woman's experience with headaches uniquely different.

Chapter 14

Headaches in children and adolescents

Children and adolescents get headaches, just like adults. In fact, some children may experience headaches before they're old enough to talk. In their school years, headaches may become common and frequent. One survey found that one-third of children who were at least 7 years old and one-half of adolescents who were at least 15 years old had headaches.

Headaches in children can be caused by common illnesses such as a cold or the flu or stress at home and school. Serious medical conditions or injuries also can lead to headaches. Yet the majority of headaches in children are primary headaches.

If the headaches persist or occur frequently, they can have a serious impact on how children interact with family and peers and perform at school. Just as with adults, treatment and understanding will help children cope better with the effects of headache. Yet children's headaches can differ from those of adults in subtle ways.

Different headaches in children

In general, children and adults get the same types of headache. If you're an adult with headaches, you may have started getting them as a child or now recognize the symptoms in your own children.

Still, not everything about the headaches experienced by children and adults are alike. Some types of headache that are more prevalent in children may become less of a problem or cease entirely as children grow older. Children's headaches also can cause physical symptoms and bodily changes not commonly seen in adults. This is especially true with migraine.

Following is a closer look at the types of headache experienced by children and how these types compare with adult headaches of the same name.

Migraine

Migraine occurs in 4 percent to 10 percent of children. Most of these children have inherited the condition. External factors such as stress, certain foods, lack of sleep or too much exertion can trigger the headaches, much as with adults. No matter what the cause, migraine may begin by or sometimes before the age of 7.

In childhood, migraine prevalence tends to be split equally between the sexes. Once puberty hits, the incidence of migraine increases notably in girls. In fact, adolescent girls are three times more likely than adolescent boys to get migraine, probably associated with the onset of menstruation.

Just like adults, child migraineurs often experience throbbing head pain, nausea, vomiting and sensitivity to light and sound during an attack. Aura — the perception of bright lights, zigzag lines and other visual disturbances before head pain begins — tends to develop around the age of 10. Yet the aura can be different from that of adults. During an aura, children may feel confused and hallucinate, their pupils may become dilated, and they may have difficulty speaking. In most cases, however, children have migraine without aura. Other common differences between migraine in adults and children include:

Pain location. Pain most often occurs on both sides of the head in children, whereas many adults experience pain on only one side. Sometimes children may experience severe abdominal pain instead of head pain.

Frequency. In general, children and adolescents get more migraine attacks than adults.

Duration. Adult migraine can last hours or even days, depending on the individual. Children's migraine can be much shorter. In children under age 15, migraine may last less than two hours and sometimes be shorter than 30 minutes.

Variation. Children, more than adults, are more likely to get migraine that is considered atypical and exhibit symptoms that can be mistaken for other ailments. These variants include:

Abdominal migraine. Although this rare migraine causes vomiting and nausea, just like common migraine, pain develops in the abdomen, not the head. As a result, young children with these headaches are often thought to have an upset stomach or the flu.

Hemiplegic migraine. Slurred speech and temporary paralysis on one side of the body — a condition known as hemiplegia — are the hallmarks of hemiplegic migraine.

Basilar-type migraine. Migraine associated with the basilar arteries — major arteries to the brain — causes severe head pain, dizziness, loss of balance, double vision, difficulty speaking, confusion and weakness. It's more common in girls than in boys.

Acute confusional migraine. This migraine, which usually occurs in adolescents, cause a sudden onset of confusion and disorientation. The symptoms last for up to 12 hours but, fortunately, these episodes are rare and resolve on their own, after a night's sleep. Later, the child may go on to develop more typical migraine. In some cases, however, a minor head injury can cause a more serious and prolonged form of this migraine.

Tension-type headache

Unlike migraine, most children do not inherit tension-type headache from their parents. Tension, stress, depression, hunger, fatigue or eyestrain can all trigger tension-type headache in children and adolescents — the same way they do in adults.

It's estimated that 15 percent of children have tension-type headache. Commonly, these headaches are episodic, causing moderate pain that is said to feel like a band of pressure tightening around the head. Children may get them from such emotional and physical stresses as staying up late to study, arguing with a family member, being teased at school or skipping a meal.

Chronic daily headache

A headache that occurs on a daily basis for months or years is known as chronic daily headache. The condition may affect up to 4 percent of adolescent girls and 2 percent of adolescent boys. Some report having a headache all the time. Others will also have episodes of more severe pain that resembles a migraine.

The reason for a chronic daily headache to develop is unclear. In most adolescents, the condition begins as episodic migraine becomes more frequent. One possible cause is the overuse of pain medication, which can result in rebound headaches.

Some children who have never had a headache before will experience the sudden onset of chronic daily headache. When this happens, it's often associated with a serious infection such as mononucleosis, a history of head trauma or another physiologic stress.

Adolescents with chronic daily headache may experience non-headache signs and symptoms as well. Many will have a sleep disorder. They may feel tired, fatigued and frustrated. Occasionally, they will also experience pain in the abdomen or back.

Cluster headache

Cluster headache is a rare form of headache. Although it's not known exactly how many children and adolescents get this type of headache, boys outnumber girls by a ratio of approximately 7 to 1. Adult males with cluster headache outnumber adult females with this headache by the same ratio.

Cluster headache is one of the most painful headaches, causing a piercing, stabbing pain behind one eye. During attacks, the pain can become so intense that children may scream or pace the room, unable to sit still. They also may appear confused or angry.

Cluster headache is classified as a headache of short duration. Attacks can last from minutes to hours and typically occur in groups (clusters). There may be multiple attacks each day or once every other day. A watery eye and runny nose accompany most attacks, and onset may take place during sleep. In contrast to a child with migraine, who may curl up under blankets in a darkened room and try to sleep, a child with a cluster headache will have a difficult time lying still with the headache.

Secondary headaches

Less than 5 percent of children's headaches are caused by disease or a physical problem. Nevertheless, the secondary causes of headache should be ruled out when head pain becomes a problem. In children, common secondary causes include the following:

Fever and infection. A headache often accompanies fever. Yet having a fever isn't necessarily bad. Fevers often help the body fight off infections. However, if children have a high temperature, headache and symptoms such as a stiff neck, weakness, seizures, sluggishness, nausea and vomiting, a serious infection of the central nervous system could be to blame. In rare cases, this could be the first signs of meningitis or encephalitis, potentially fatal infections that require immediate medical attention (see Chapter 12).

Seventy percent of the people who get meningitis are children under age 5, but the incidence of the disease is increasing among young people between the ages of 15 and 24. One form of encephalitis is associated with such viral infections as chickenpox, measles or mumps. In older children, the initial symptoms may be a severe headache and sensitivity to light.

Head trauma. A bump on the head, even a relatively minor blow, can quickly result in a headache. Although tests are needed to determine if the child has a concussion or brain injury, certain signs and symptoms may be cause for concern. If a child experiences dizziness, confusion, fatigue or memory loss in addition to headache following head trauma, contact your doctor immediately.

Brain tumor. A brain tumor is rarely the cause of headaches in children. Still, a tumor can develop at an early age. Be aware if a child has headaches that progressively worsen, are always in the same location, awaken him or her from sleep or are worse in the morning. If the headaches are accompanied by nausea, vomiting or blurred vision, contact your doctor as soon as possible.

Idiopathic intracranial hypertension. This medical condition, also called pseudotumor cerebri, is a result of increased fluid pressure within the skull. It can lead to a persistent headache, double vision, nausea and vomiting, and swelling of the optic nerve. Children taking medications such as tetracyclines and corticosteroids or high doses of vitamins, particularly vitamin A, may be susceptible to this condition. Children with frequent sinus or ear infections also may become predisposed. Pressure within the skull is relieved either with a lumbar puncture or a diuretic.

Dental problems. Children who regularly grind or clench their teeth while sleeping (a condition called bruxism, pronounced BRUK-siz-uhm) or have problems with their temporomandibular joint, which joins the jawbone to the skull, can develop headaches. Bruxism occurs in as many as one in three children, often around the ages of five and six, and in most cases the children outgrow the problem. Children who complain of jaw or face pain along with a headache may have a temporomandibular disorder, which includes misaligned bones in the jaw and skull or poorly fitting braces.

Chiari malformation. Chiari (kee-AH-ree) malformation is a rare disorder in which part of the brain protrudes through an opening in the back of the skull. This condition may or may not be apparent at birth. Adolescents unaware that they have the malformation may develop headaches located in the back of the head that occur with coughing or sneezing. Other problems may include difficulty with swallowing, curvature of the spine (scoliosis) and back pain. This malformation can be treated possibly with surgery.

Diagnosis

Children too young to verbalize their discomfort may cry, turn pale, vomit or bang their heads when they experience head pain. If you think your child's discomfort could be related to an illness or injury, it's important to seek medical attention. But not all headaches require a trip to the doctor. In fact, a child with an occasional migraine or tension-type headache may need little more than some quiet time, a few hours sleep and an over-the-counter pain reliever (at child strength). When headaches become more chronic in nature or begin to disrupt school performance, extracurricular activities, or family life, your child may require more aggressive treatment.

A medical evaluation generally is recommended when a child begins having new or persistent headaches. Doctors will likely make the diagnosis after they take a detailed history of the headaches and perform a neurological exam, which tests such functions as memory, concentration, vision, hearing, balance and coordination. Some doctors may ask the family to keep a headache diary, noting times and places that headaches occur, as well as any emotions or behaviors that accompany the headaches. This can provide the doctors with information they'll need to identify possible triggers of the headaches.

Additional tests may be required, especially when secondary causes of headache are suspected. These tests may include everything from a blood test to check for infection to magnetic resonance imaging (MRI) to look for abnormalities in the brain.

Treatment

Once a diagnosis is made, headache treatment can be customized for an individual child or adolescent. In general, primary headaches in children are treated with a combination of drug and non-drug therapies. Many children respond well to this approach.

Establishing good eating and sleeping habits and making time for relaxation and regular exercise are key strategies for keeping headaches from becoming a chronic problem. Indeed, common headache triggers in children and adolescents include skipping meals and not getting enough sleep.

A related problem for many children is overscheduling. Headaches may worsen as the school year progresses, even though the children appear to be enjoying and excelling at school, because their free time is swallowed up by homework and activities.

Like adults, many children benefit from avoiding specific foods and food additives that trigger their headaches. These may include monosodium glutamate, nitrates, chocolates and cheeses. An occasional child will get headaches from exercise or extreme heat. It's important to recognize the influence of these factors on headache, as we're able to control our exposure to many of them.

If nondrug therapies aren't enough to reduce the frequency or alleviate the pain of primary headaches, the use of pain relievers at the time a headache starts may become part of the treatment plan.

It's important to treat head pain as early as possible. The longer a headache goes untreated, the less effective a pain reliever will be. It's also important to use a dose of medicine that's appropriate for children. Specific doses can be discussed with your doctor.

Medications for treating children's headaches can be categorized into three groups:

Over-the-counter medication to relieve acute pain. These medications include analgesics such as acetaminophen (Tylenol, others), ibuprofen (Advil, Motrin, others) and naproxen (Aleve, Naprosyn, others). When taken early, they're typically effective. Don't give aspirin and combination drugs containing aspirin to children under 16 years of age because aspirin has been linked to Reye's syndrome, a rare but potentially life-threatening condition.

Prescription medication to relieve severe headaches. Although triptan medications still are under review by the Food and Drug Administration (FDA) for use in children, early studies have shown them to be safe and effective in 12- to 18-year-olds. As a result, triptans now are being used more as off-label drugs (drugs used for a purpose or in a way that does not have FDA approval), especially in teens. Antiemetic drugs, used to treat the nausea and vomiting that can accompany migraine, also may be an option. They include promethazine (Phenergan), trimethobenzamide (Tigan) and prochlorperazine (Compazine).

Prescription medication to prevent frequent headaches. If a child has two or more severe headaches a week, he or she may take a daily medication intended to prevent headaches. These medications include tricyclic antidepressants, beta blockers, calcium channel blockers, serotonin agonists, antihistamines and anti-seizure drugs. Like the triptan medications, these drugs still are under review by the FDA for use in children and teens. Yet a number are being used off-label in children.

Drug precautions

Medication strategies will depend on the individual child and the type of headache. No matter what the medication, certain precautions are necessary for all children taking an over-the-counter or prescription medication. These precautions include:

Reading labels carefully. Use only the dosage recommended for children. Some over-the-counter products come in infant, child and adult strengths but may look the same. If you're confused about dosages based on a child's weight or age, ask a doctor or pharmacist for help. Also, heed any warning that states a product is not to be given to children.

Limiting the use of pain relievers. Too much reliance on pain medication often causes rebound headaches. Generally, try to use medication no more than twice a week.

Asking about possible side effects. Although many drugs are used to treat headaches in children, not all have been officially approved for children by the FDA. Be sure to ask if a drug has been studied in your child's age range and what side effects might occur. Also, check with your doctor before giving your child alternative headache treatments such as vitamins or herbal remedies.

Scheduling follow-up exams to evaluate treatment. If medications aren't working effectively, your doctor may need to change the type or dosage of a drug. Once headaches are under control, preventive medications sometimes can be withdrawn under the doctor's supervision.

Psychological issues

Headaches are much more than a physical problem. Children and adolescents who frequently miss school, avoid foods that other kids enjoy or skip social activities because of headaches may feel different and isolated from their peers. Headache symptoms such as vomiting, dizziness and blurred vision — any of which may come on suddenly — can draw unwanted attention to your child. This can make him or her feel reluctant to be away from home or anxious in an unknown or peer-packed environment.

Indeed, studies show that headaches can hinder academic performance and emotional development. The following can help children cope with psychological issues related to headaches:

Encourage communication. A child may not feel so alone if given a chance to express his or her concerns. Talk with your child about what it feels like to have a headache. Make your child aware of other family members who have headaches. It can be reassuring to learn that he or she is not so different from everyone else. Keeping a headache journal also can help your child feel more in control and understand what may be triggering the pain.

Partner with teachers and health professionals. Let school officials know when headaches are interfering with your child's attendance or performance in class. School officials can be major allies if your child requires medication during the day or needs treatment as soon as the symptoms begin. Once your child is aware that teachers understand the situation, he or she may worry less about what to do if a headache develops during school hours.

Maintain proper focus. Although it's important not to ignore the physical and emotional toll that headaches can take, try not to let the condition rule your child's life or be used as an excuse for not participating and achieving. Head pain may be a legitimate reason for missing school or skipping chores, but don't let it become a way to get attention or avoid responsibilities. Instead, teach your child the best ways to prevent bad days and make the most of good ones.

Consider counseling. If headaches interfere too much with daily life, you may want to take your child to see a counselor. Individual counseling can help your child learn to deal with issues that may be keeping him or her from going to school, connecting with peers or participating in family life. Family counseling also may help parents or siblings who have developed feelings of guilt, fear or resentment toward a child with headaches.

Taking control

If headaches are a problem, a family physician or pediatrician should be able to help develop a treatment plan for your child. But even with treatment, not all children will stop having headaches. In fact, like adults, children may have to try different strategies before finding adequate relief from pain. With proper support, headaches don't have to be a major interference in your child's life.

Chapter 15

Older adults and headaches

As you get older, the aches and pains in your muscles and joints only seem to increase. But the opposite tends to be true with those headaches that have bothered you for so many years. Migraine and other primary headaches that were common when you were a young adult may ease and become less of a problem with age.

Still, you can't count on the headaches to disappear completely. Primary headaches that seem to have always been part of your life may continue to occur in some form. On occasion, new primary headaches may develop that you'd never had before. Of greater concern to older adults are secondary headaches, which become more common as you age because of the increased occurrence of medical conditions that may cause pain.

Furthermore, for older adults, the growing number of health concerns may complicate existing headache treatments. Some pain medications that you could take before may not be tolerated as well now because your body's metabolism has slowed. Other pain medications may not be safe to take at the same time you're using drugs for other medical problems. As a result, your headache treatment may have to be adjusted, making greater use of mild or low-dose medications, nondrug therapies or medications primarily designed for other conditions.

Prevalence of primary headaches

Although headaches know no age boundaries, once you're past the age of 50, headaches typically become less frequent and less severe. Indeed, studies show the percentage of men and women who have headaches decreases significantly as they get older. For example, researchers in one study found that 92 percent of women and 74 percent of men between the ages of 21 and 34 had headaches. This percentage dropped to 66 percent of women and 53 percent of men between the ages of 55 and 74. Percentages dropped even lower after age 75.

Despite this decrease, headaches still pose problems for some individuals well into old age. As in other age groups, primary headaches account for the majority of headaches in older adults. Most often, the headaches represent a continuation of an existing condition. In some cases, however, primary headaches can occur for the first time after age 50, or different signs and symptoms may develop that can raise suspicions about a secondary cause.

Migraine

The frequency of headache attacks begins to decline gradually for many people with migraine when they reach their 40s. If someone hasn't had migraine by age 50, he or she is less likely to ever have one afterward. Only 2 percent of adults develop migraine after reaching this age.

Migraine typically causes a throbbing or pounding head pain that can last for hours or days, and often it's accompanied by symptoms such as nausea and vomiting (See Chapter 4). It also may be preceded by aura. As you age, the severity of migraine may lessen, and aura may become less common.

If you had migraine with aura as a younger adult, however, you may continue to develop the aura — even though head pain has almost disappeared. In fact, in this type of late-life migraine, head-ache pain is present only 50 percent of the time and may be of only mild intensity. Late-life migraine can also be accompanied by blurred vision, numbness or tingling in the arms or legs, dizziness and speech difficulties.

When head pain doesn't follow aura, it's advisable to see your doctor. Although nothing may be wrong, it's wise to rule out other conditions that could be to blame for the signs and symptoms you're having. A primary concern is transient ischemic attack (TIA), a temporary decrease in blood supply to part of your brain and the warning sign of a possible stroke to follow.

Most TIAs last for just a few minutes although the signs and symptoms may continue for up to 24 hours. Late-life migraine attacks, on the other hand, tend to last longer, and one or more symptoms may end before other symptoms begin. Episodes of this migraine may occur regularly. Nevertheless, an evaluation by your doctor is recommended. If TIA is to blame, treatment will focus on improving blood supply to the brain to prevent a later stroke. If migraine is the problem, your doctor may prescribe preventive medication, especially if attacks occur frequently.

Tension-type headache

Like migraine, tension-type headache may occur less frequently as you get older. But this type of headache is the most common headache among older adults. In fact, 10 percent of older adults experience a tension-type headache for the first time after age 50.

Because tension-type headache is commonly associated with the stress of work, school or parenting, it may seem odd to experience this headache just when you thought the pace of life was slowing down. Yet retirement, the loss of a loved one, a medical illness or other major life change can produce the kind of stress that triggers tension-type headache (See Chapter 9).

Most often, tension-type headache feels as though a band of pressure is tightening around your head, and the pain may last for hours or days. If it's new or begins to occur with more frequency, it's best to contact your doctor. Headaches that occur more than a few times a week, for instance, could mean you're experiencing rebound headaches from medication overuse. Depression, arthritis of the neck, thyroid disorders and other medical conditions also may cause head pain. Whether the headache is associated with a secondary disorder or not, there's no reason to endure pain. Medications can relieve or prevent the attacks.

Cluster headache

Cluster headache is uncommon, but this painful disorder is most prevalent in adults between 20 and 50 years of age. Still, you may continue to have bouts of the headache when you're past the age of 50, or even develop a more chronic form of the headache. Although rare, cluster headache also may occur for the first time in an older adult, even after age 70.

Cluster headache causes a stabbing or piercing pain in or around one eye or the temple area and may last from 45 to 90 minutes on average. As the name implies, the headache attacks cluster together, occurring during periods generally lasting from six to 12 weeks, followed by periods of time with no headache. An attack is often accompanied by a red or teary eye and runny nose on the same side as the head pain (See Chapter 10).

Any change in the pattern of your cluster periods should be brought to the attention of your doctor, even if it seems to be improvement. Also, review your treatment options, as some treatments may require more careful monitoring as you age.

Hypnic headache

Hypnic headache is the only primary headache that occurs almost exclusively among older adults. These headaches have been reported in men and women in their 40s. However, most people experience their first hypnic headache between ages 65 and 85.

A hypnic headache occurs at night and wakes you up from sleep, often striking at the same hour each evening. The throbbing pain is moderate to severe and of short duration, typically lasting from 15 minutes to one or two hours. Migraine and cluster headache also can awaken you from sleep, but they rarely happen exclusively during the nighttime.

Some conditions that occur in older adults regularly cause nighttime headaches. They include cranial arteritis, sleep apnea, brain tumor and subdural hematoma (See Chapter 12). As a result, secondary causes of head pain typically must be ruled out before hypnic headache can be diagnosed. A dose of caffeine at bedtime may prevent an attack. Treatment usually involves medications such as lithium carbonate or indomethacin.

Secondary headache disorders

In children and young adults, primary headaches account for more than 90 percent of all headaches. In adults over age 50, that percentage drops to 66 percent, while the percentage of secondary headaches rises. In fact, once you're over the age of 65, the risk of a serious secondary disorder causing head pain increases 10 times that for younger groups.

Although not all headaches are cause for alarm, new headaches or changes in the usual headache patterns are often warning signs, especially for older adults. Indeed, diseases and conditions that are common in adults over age 50 typically make the list of most likely causes for headaches whenever the head pain seems out of the ordinary. These medical problems may include:

Cerebrovascular disease

As you age, you're at greater risk of conditions that narrow, clog, inflame or injure your blood vessels, obstructing the flow of blood to your brain. A prolonged interruption of blood flow can be life-threatening or lead to brain damage. Even brief disruptions in flow can decrease brain function and cause headaches and problems with vision, speech or mental capabilities. Pain may vary, depending on the type and severity of the condition:

High blood pressure. About 50 million Americans have high blood pressure, but many don't realize they do. That's because for most people there are no obvious signs and symptoms of the disease that would signal a problem. Dull headaches may occur at the back of the head in early stages, but more often, headaches don't appear until blood pressure has reached an extremely high level and possibly damaged blood vessels or vital organs. The cause of this condition isn't always known, but certain factors, such as age, increase your risk.

Transient ischemic attack and stroke. A transient ischemic attack (TIA) is sometimes called a ministroke or stroke warning because it momentarily disrupts blood flow to your brain and increases the risk of stroke. Strokes typically interrupt blood supply for a longer period of time and can damage your brain.

Both TIAs and strokes may happen when fatty deposits that collect on the walls of your arteries block blood flow. Headaches may occur before, after or during TIAs and strokes. Onset can occur gradually or suddenly and may be accompanied by weakness in your arms or legs, numbness or tingling, difficulty speaking, a decrease in or loss of vision, and a loss of balance and coordination. Old age, high blood pressure, heart disease, diabetes and smoking all increase your risk of TIAs and stroke.

Cranial arteritis. This condition, also known as giant cell arteritis or temporal arteritis, almost exclusively affects older adults. In fact, the average age of onset is 70. Inflamed arteries cause throbbing head pain, scalp tenderness and jaw pain. Diminished blood flow to your eyes or brain can provoke complications such as blindness or stroke. The cause of cranial arteritis is unknown, but you're at greater risk if you're an older female of Northern European descent. Rheumatoid arthritis and an arthritic condition of the neck, shoulders and hips known as polymyalgia rheumatica also increase your risk. Treatment often involves a corticosteroid such as prednisone (Deltasone, Sterapred).

Intracranial disorders

Brain tumors are a relatively rare cause of headaches. But the formation of these abnormal cell clusters becomes more common in old age and can produce new or more severe headaches by putting pressure on the brain. In fact, head pain often is the first sign of a tumor developing. Dull, achy headaches may begin in the morning, or they may disrupt your sleep at night. Over time, however, the pain worsens, accompanied by other signs and symptoms such as nausea, vomiting, blurred or double vision, balance problems and speech difficulties.

A steady or fluctuating headache could be the result of a subdural hematoma, which also puts pressure on your brain. If you're an older adult, these hematomas can occur spontaneously. But head injuries from accidents or falls are the most frequent cause. The condition is more likely in adults with age-related brain atrophy (shrinkage). The use of blood thinning medications and chronic alcohol use also may increase the risk.

Neuralgias

Trigeminal neuralgia, which occurs primarily after age 50, involves searing bursts of facial pain that may strike unexpectedly. The condition is caused by a disruption of the trigeminal nerve, which carries sensation from areas of your face to your brain. Attacks can last from a few seconds to about a minute and may be brought on by talking, brushing your teeth, shaving, putting on makeup, or any other form of facial stimulation (see Chapter 11).

Postherpetic neuralgia is another neuralgia that becomes more common with age. The condition is a complication of shingles, which occurs when a past chickenpox virus is reactivated inside your nerve cells. A sharp, burning or aching pain remains in the affected areas, such as the face, long after the shingles rash has healed. Not everyone who has shingles will develop postherpetic neuralgia, but you're more likely to get it as an older adult.

Conditions of the neck, eyes and jaw

Dull, persistent headaches, particularly at the back of the head, may be caused by cervical spondylosis (spon-duh-LOH-sis), a disorder caused by abnormal wear on the cartilage and bones of your neck and compression of one or more nerve roots. The greatest risk factor of spondylosis is aging. X-rays reveal signs of degeneration of the cervical spine in 70 percent of women and 85 percent of men by age 60, indicating that many older adults may have or will develop cervical spondylosis.

Glaucoma is an eye disease affecting about 3 million Americans, mostly over the age of 50. Several types of glaucoma exist, but all cause increased pressure inside the eyeball that damages the optic nerve. In acute angle-closure glaucoma, sudden, severe pain, usually behind one eye, may develop into a generalized headache.

Headaches that accompany jaw tenderness, a dull ache in front of your ears and a clicking or grating sound when you open your mouth could mean a problem with your temporomandibular joints. These joints connect your lower jawbone to your skull. Pain and tenderness can spread from the temporomandibular joints as a result of wear and tear, arthritic inflammation, injury, stress or poorly fitting dentures.

Metabolic disorders

Metabolic disorders such as hyperthyroidism and hypothyroidism cause an imbalance in the hormones that control many body functions, resulting in fatigue, weakness, nausea and head pain. Headache also may be a symptom of hyperparathyroidism, a condition that affects the levels of certain minerals in your blood and bones. Diabetes, high blood pressure and certain kidney diseases can lead to problems such as chronic kidney failure or end-stage kidney disease. Damaged kidneys are associated with a number of symptoms, including headaches.

Medication side effects and overuse

Many diseases and conditions that are common in old age require medications that can cause mild or moderate headaches. In fact, headaches are a common side effect of medications prescribed for high blood pressure, heart disease, emphysema, ulcers, depression, Parkinson's disease and menopause. Over-the-counter drugs such as analgesics and decongestants also can be a source of chronic head pain — especially if you overuse them. This type of daily

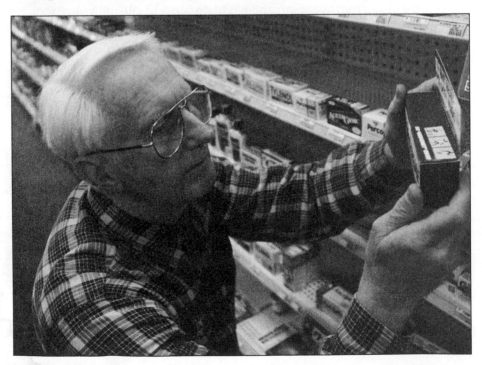

head pain is known as rebound headaches because they occur (rebound) when the effect of medication wears off (see Chapter 9 for more detail). Older adults, who often take multiple medications for chronic illnesses and conditions, may be particularly prone to this type of headache.

Modifications to treatment

If you develop a type of headache after age 50 that you've never had before or detect changes in the pattern of headaches that you've had for years, it's advisable to see your doctor. Although there may be no cause for worry, it's important to review your current headache treatments to find the best and safest way to relieve or prevent head pain.

If you have an occasional migraine or tension-type headache, taking over-the-counter pain relievers at the first sign of head pain is generally the best way to dull or stop the headache. If the headache is more frequent or more difficult to treat, however, certain medications may need to be limited or replaced with alternatives because of potential complications related to your age, your overall medical condition, or both.

Overusing over-the-counter drugs such as aspirin, ibuprofen and naproxen can cause nausea, stomach pain, stomach bleeding or ulcers, particularly for older adults, for whom these drugs can be more toxic. Pain relievers that combine acetaminophen with a more powerful barbiturate or opiate drug are closely associated with rebound headaches.

Prescription medications designed specifically to ease the pain of migraine or other chronic headaches may present other complications. Some of these medications work by constricting blood vessels. But reducing blood flow to the head and heart can be dangerous if you have a medical condition that may already be narrowing the blood vessels. As a result, these drugs usually aren't recommended if you have or are at high risk of a number of conditions that are common among older adults, including high blood pressure, stroke and coronary artery disease.

Corticosteroids, which are used to relieve migraine and cluster headache, may no longer be an option for older adults. They can have serious side effects such as ulcers or an increase in blood pressure. The long-term use of these drugs also can cause eye diseases such as glaucoma or cataracts and lower your immune system, making you more likely to develop infections.

Still, these restrictions don't mean you'll be living in pain. Lower doses of pain-relieving drugs can be combined with nondrug therapies such as stress management and relaxation therapy to help lessen the severity of headaches when they occur.

Some medications used to treat other health conditions, such as high blood pressure, depression and epilepsy, may be used to prevent different types of headache. These medications include beta blockers, tricyclic antidepressants and anti-seizure drugs. However, doses typically start at low levels and increased gradually to see how your body reacts. That's because as you get older, it becomes more difficult for your body to process and eliminate medications. Pre-existing health problems, such as asthma, diabetes and heart disease, also may limit your use of these drugs or eliminate them as an option altogether. (For more information on preventive medications, see Chapter 6.)

Newer pain medications designed to cause fewer side effects offer more options for older adults. For instance, COX-2 inhibitors such as celecoxib (Celebrex) and rofecoxib (Vioxx) may provide the relief of aspirin or ibuprofen with lower risk of stomach and stomach lining damage. Additional research is needed to verify this benefit and to test the long-term effects of this drug.

In recent years, nondrug therapies such as massage and acupuncture have gained popularity as complements to more conventional headache treatment, particularly for individuals who have medical conditions that prohibit or limit medications. Before using any treatment, consult with your doctor to find the option that's best for your age and overall health.

Chapter 16

Complementary and alternative therapies

If you've sought help for headaches in recent years, you know that prescription and nonprescription medications top the list of treatments. But more and more people are willing to consider options outside the mainstream of conventional medical practice. One recent study of people seeking treatment for headaches found that almost 85 percent of those surveyed had tried a complementary or alternative therapy.

The National Center for Complementary and Alternative Medicine, a division of the National Institutes of Health (NIH), defines complementary medicine as unconventional treatments used *in addition to* treatments recommended by your physician. An example might be getting a massage to ease muscle tension as well as using pain medication. Alternative medicine includes treatments used *in place of* traditional medicine. This might mean substituting herbal products for a common pain reliever.

Many complementary and alternative therapies have been in use for years and are a welcome option for those people who experience side effects from medications, have other conditions that restrict medication use or are not getting enough relief from medications alone. But not all nondrug therapies have been studied as headache treatments, and others require additional study, leaving open questions about their effectiveness and safety.

Evaluating treatment options

Complementary and alternative treatments may expand your options for pain relief. Yet sorting through the pros and cons of these therapies can be confusing. If you're considering one of these treatments, think about these guidelines:

Gather information about the treatment. The Internet is ideal for keeping up with the latest on complementary and alternative treatments. Unfortunately, the Internet can also be a source of misinformation. Web sites created by the major medical centers, national organizations, universities and government organizations are the most reliable. A good place to start is the National Center for Complementary and Alternative Medicine (*www.nccam.nih.gov*).

Find and evaluate treatment providers. Check your state government listings for agencies that regulate and license health providers. Your doctor, another health care professional and people who have received the treatment you're considering can be a good sources of information.

Consider treatment cost. Many complementary and alternative therapies are not covered by health insurance. Find out exactly how much the treatment will cost and whether your health insurance will pay for at least a part of it.

Check your attitude. Strike a balance between being open-minded and skeptical. In other words, stay open to various treatments but evaluate them carefully.

Opt for complementary over alternative medicine. Research indicates that unconventional medical treatments are most commonly used to complement rather than replace conventional care. Ideally, various forms of treatment should work together. You don't want to ignore a treatment that's proved to be effective, replacing it with one that may or may not help.

This chapter provides an overview of common complementary and alternative therapies, such as massage, hypnosis, acupuncture, chiropractic care, and herbal remedies, focusing on what evidence is available on their usefulness as headache treatments.

Manipulation and touch

The attraction of certain complementary and alternative treatments for some people is that they involve human touch. Examples include chiropractic treatment, massage, acupuncture and electrical stimulation. These therapies are based on the manipulation or movement of one or more body parts.

Chiropractic treatment

Chiropractic medicine is perhaps the most common complementary therapy in the United States. Care is based on the belief that certain conditions, such as chronic pain, result from an impairment of your nervous system due to problems with your joints and especially your spine. Chiropractic, which literally means "done by hand," involves manipulating, stretching and adjusting joints or vertebrae to relieve the impairment of your nerves. Although chiropractors can't prescribe drugs or perform surgery, their services increasingly are covered by medical insurance. They sometimes work in association with medical doctors.

Spinal manipulation can effectively treat uncomplicated low back pain. However, studies don't fully support claims that chiropractic also relieves headaches. Pursuing this therapy should be undertaken with care because chiropractic manipulation of the neck sometimes can increase spinal pain and, very rarely, damage the vertebral arteries, which may lead to headaches.

Massage

Massage involves the manipulation of your body's soft tissues. Massage therapists use their hands primarily to knead muscles and tendons that are stiff and sore. The procedure is often included in physical therapy and nursing care to relieve muscle tension or promote relaxation in people undergoing other types of medical treatment. Massage can be used to improve range of motion in joints and increase production of the body's natural painkillers.

Although the effectiveness of massage as a headache treatment hasn't been determined fully, the procedure is generally considered safe. It can loosen tight, tender muscles in the back of your head, neck and shoulders that may contribute to headaches. Massage also can be an effective way to relieve stress and tension.

Any type of massage should relax you. If you feel pain or discomfort during the procedure, speak up immediately. Also, avoid getting a massage over an open wound, skin infection, inflamed joint, or area of weakened bone or thrombophlebitis (a blood clot and inflammation in a vein).

Acupuncture

Acupuncture, a technique that has existed for more than 2,500 years, has become one of the most accepted forms of complementary and alternative medicine. The National Institutes of Health has concluded that acupuncture can play a useful role in controlling headaches and other conditions that cause chronic pain.

The philosophical basis of this therapy is that your health depends on the free circulation of blood and a subtle energy called chi (pronounced chee). Chi flows through your body along 14 pathways called meridians. When the flow of chi is interrupted, illness results. Inserting hair-thin needles under the skin at specific points along the meridians is thought to remove blockages and restore a healthy balance to your body. Studies indicate that acupuncture may work, in part, by promoting the release of natural painkillers and other chemicals in the central nervous system.

During a typical session, an acupuncturist inserts anywhere from one to 20 needles into your skin for 15 to 30 minutes, depending on the condition you're being treated for. There should be little or no pain from insertion of the needles. You'll probably require several sessions to get results. If nothing's happening after six or eight sessions, acupuncture is probably not for you.

Adverse side effects from acupuncture are rare, but can occur. Make sure your acupuncturist is experienced and practices good hygiene, including the use of sterile needles.

Electrical stimulation

Transcutaneous electrical nerve stimulation (TENS) is intended to relieve pain by preventing pain signals from reaching your brain. In the procedure, small electrodes are placed on your skin near painful areas. The electrodes are attached to a battery-powered stimulator that you wear. The stimulator delivers mild impulses through the electrodes, helping to reduce pain.

Just how this procedure relieves pain isn't clear. One theory holds that the impulses block nerve pathways that carry pain messages to the brain. Another theory suggests that TENS triggers the release of pain-reducing chemicals called endorphins in your central nervous system.

TENS works best for acute back and neck pain. It has been less successful for chronic pain, although some people with a chronic condition do appear to benefit from it. Studies of TENS as a treatment for headaches offer mixed results. Most often, TENS is used along with exercise and other pain therapies.

A similar treatment called percutaneous electronic nerve stimulation (PENS) is now under study for pain relief. Like TENS, this therapy delivers an electric impulse to your nerves. But PENS delivers the current through thin, acupuncture-like needles that penetrate your skin.

Mind-Body Connection

Treatments in this category are based on the idea that your mind and body are inextricably linked. Negative thoughts and feelings can produce symptoms in your body. Treatment aims to help you to detach from these thoughts and feelings or to actively change them. Often, one of these techniques is combined with another therapy to bring about relief.

Hypnosis

Hypnosis has long been crowd-pleasing entertainment. But it's more than just a magic trick. Reports indicate that hypnosis has been used as a migraine treatment for more than a century. In recent years, several studies have shown that weekly hypnosis sessions can reduce the severity and frequency of tension-type headache. The use of this form of therapy to manage pain has gained support from the NIH.

Hypnosis involves entering a state of deep relaxation while keeping your mind alert and open to suggestion. During a session, an expert might suggest ways to decrease your perception of pain and increase your ability to cope with it. A typical suggestion might be to visualize a place that you think of as safe and calm.

The success of hypnosis depends on the expertise of the practitioner and on your willingness to participate. If you show resistance, you may not be able to be hypnotized, even by a trained professional. If you're open to the idea, you may eventually be able to develop the skills to hypnotize yourself.

Professional hypnotists and occasionally psychiatrists and psychologists practice hypnosis. But be careful to ask for credentials and to check references, because hypnosis is a poorly regulated field. At the same time, don't worry about what you see in movies and on television. Even under hypnosis, you can't be forced to do something that's truly against your will.

Meditation

Meditation is a way to calm your mind and body. Its origins can be traced to various religious and cultural traditions. Hundreds of studies have been published about the potential benefits of various forms of meditation, and while the quality of these studies is uneven, they do suggest grounds for further research.

During meditation you sit quietly and focus on a simple activity, such as breathing, or on a single word or phrase that's repeated many times. You may find this practice creates a deeply restful state in which your breathing slows and your muscles relax. The ensuing relaxation may help you manage pain and reduce stress that can trigger or worsen a headache.

Yoga

Yoga represents a spiritual path for some people and a way to promote physical flexibility, strength and endurance for others. In America, the term *yoga* generally is associated with one particular school of this ancient discipline — hatha yoga — that combines gentle breathing exercises and meditation with movement, through a series of postures called asanas. There are only a few recent studies of yoga in medical literature, some of which suggest that it may help you cope with pain. In any case, yoga is likely to help you relax and manage stress and unlikely to be harmful.

To be effective, yoga requires discipline, concentration and regular practice. You can find qualified instructors at yoga schools or learn on your own through books and videotapes. An instructor may be able to adapt postures to your level of flexibility.

Dietary Supplements

Walk down the aisles of most pharmacies or grocery stores and you'll likely find a section with various complementary or alternative remedies claiming to treat many common ailments, including headaches. The vitamin, mineral and herb products displayed in this section are all designated dietary supplements by the Food and Drug Administration (FDA).

These supplements are popularly thought of as "natural" and therefore less dangerous than prescription drugs. But often, little scientific evidence exists to support or refute this notion since supplements aren't subject to the same rigorous testing and quality control as drugs. In fact, the Dietary Supplement Health and Education Act, which was passed in 1994, limited the FDA's control over products labeled dietary supplements. The act stated that manufacturers don't have to prove to the FDA that a product is safe or effective before it goes on the market. Even so, an increasing number of supplements are now under study.

Vitamins and minerals
In general, the effectiveness of vitamins and minerals for treating acute headaches is not supported by scientific research. But studies indicate that magnesium, riboflavin and coenzyme Q-10 may be somewhat helpful in preventing migraine.

Magnesium. Your body needs the mineral magnesium for bone building and the proper function of nerves and muscles. You get magnesium in your diet from foods such as dark green leafy vegetables, whole grain cereals and breads, seafood, legumes and nuts.

Precautions when using supplements

If you're considering using supplements to treat headaches, check with your doctor. Some supplements may interfere with the effectiveness of prescription or over-the-counter drugs or have other harmful effects.

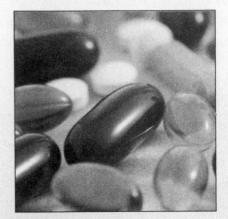

Also, read the label carefully for dosing directions. The quality and strength of supplements can vary greatly by brand. Look for the letters USP (United States Pharmacopoeia) or NF (National Formulary), which indicate the supplements meet certain standards of quality.

Studies show that some people with migraine also have low levels of magnesium. Other studies indicate that magnesium supplements, taken orally, work as a preventive treatment for migraine.

Riboflavin. Riboflavin, also known as vitamin B-2, is necessary for the growth and repair of your body's tissues. Dietary sources of riboflavin include milk and dairy products, liver, fish and other seafood. Study results show that people taking large doses of the vitamin had significantly fewer migraine attacks than those taking a placebo. These doses of riboflavin did not offer acute pain relief. According to researchers, the vitamin may need to be used for several months before benefits occur.

Coenzyme Q-10. Unlike vitamin B-2, your body produces coenzyme Q-10. But you can also find the coenzyme in foods such as salmon, mackerel, spinach and soybeans, and you can buy it as a supplement. CoQ-10, as it's called, is being studied as a treatment for cancer and heart disease. In addition, research indicates that CoQ-10 may be useful in treating headaches. In one study, there was a significant improvement in the frequency and duration of episodic migraine attacks among participants taking Co-Q10, enough so to warrant further research.

Herbal remedies

Several herbal remedies have been reported to help treat headaches. Much of this information is based on anecdotal or unverified evidence. But some herbs have been tested to determine their effectiveness as a headache treatment.

Studies indicate feverfew, a plant in the chrysanthemum family, may reduce the frequency and severity of migraine because of an active ingredient called parthenolide. Feverfew products vary widely in the amount of parthenolide they contain. If you're using blood thinners such as aspirin or warfarin (Coumadin), avoid feverfew, which inhibits clotting in your bloodstream. Also, don't take feverfew if you're pregnant.

Another herbal remedy that has helped in the treatment of migraine is butterbur, a perennial shrub that has been used medicinally for centuries. Side effects may include stomach upset, diarrhea and a form of hepatitis. You may hear anecdotal reports of other herbal remedies for headaches, such as ginger and ginkgo. Even if you hear positive testimonials, it pays to be cautious when taking any herbal medicines because these treatments can interact with other medications or cause side effects.

Other options

Other complementary and alternative treatments have been promoted for pain management. Before you try any of them, be sure to read the sidebar "Evaluating treatment options" in this chapter.

Aromatherapy

This ancient form of healing uses essential oils — oils having concentrated odors or flavors of the plants from which they're derived. These oils are believed to help treat various conditions, including chronic pain, when massaged into your skin or inhaled. Peppermint and eucalyptus oils, in particular, have been found to relieve tension-type headache. A potential problem involves the strong odors of certain oils that, in some individuals, trigger a migraine or increase nausea that accompanies a headache.

Music therapy

Practitioners of music therapy claim that performing or listening to music can lower stress, reduce symptoms of depression and provide pain relief. Music therapy hasn't been researched extensively, and studies that have been published show mixed results. But music therapy poses few risks and is inexpensive to try.

Although many complementary and alternative treatments have a long history, it's not clear how effective some of them are for treating headache pain. While some therapies have gained mainstream acceptance, others haven't been adequately studied.

If you decide to use an unconventional treatment for headache, take time to evaluate the possible benefits and risks before trying it. Make sure to let your doctor know about any and all therapies you're using. These days, many doctors are open to treatments that complement mainstream medical practice. And they can help protect your health by alerting you to possible dangers that an unconventional therapy may pose.

Chapter 17

Living with headache

The impact of headaches extends beyond the hours of pain. Chronic or severe headaches can take a tremendous toll on your confidence and self-esteem. You may struggle to finish daily chores at home and meet deadlines at work. You may face misunderstandings or lack of sympathy from family members, friends, co-workers and supervisors.

As challenging as it is to live with headaches, there's cause for optimism. Many people with chronic headaches enjoy productive lives, and there's no reason why you can't be one of them. Your goal is to gain a sense of control over your headaches. Having confidence that you can cope your condition is half the battle.

Finding support

Frequent headaches can rob you of the desire to stay socially connected. When your head is throbbing, the last place you want to be is around other people. It can be difficult for others to understand what you're going through. It's easy to feel isolated.

A way to avoid isolation is to seek companionship and guidance from others. Health care professionals, family, friends and colleagues can support your efforts. Studies show that people with a

solid support system have many advantages in maintaining their
health. They are better able to cope with chronic pain, are less likely
to experience depression, are more independent, recover faster
from illness and live longer.

Building a support network starts with finding a doctor who
understands your condition and helps you develop an effective
treatment plan. Friends and family can be informed of the best
ways to assist you. Some people find it helpful to join a support
group, while others relate well to a therapist or counselor. The bottom line is, you don't have to do it all on your own.

Your doctor

A key to coping with headaches is finding the right doctor. In your
relationship with a doctor, there must be mutual trust, honesty and
commitment. Look for someone who is knowledgeable about headaches, listens well and encourages questions, makes you feel at ease
and may be open to multiple treatment strategies, including medication, exercise and stress management.

If your doctor isn't motivated to work with you, consider looking for another health care professional. Before selecting a new doctor, check with your health insurance provider to make sure that
the care will be covered under your policy.

Family and friends

Your family and friends can provide invaluable assistance as you
learn to live with chronic headaches. Many people say that the family members who also get headaches are their most helpful allies.
But reliance on family and friends requires communication and
patience on both sides.

As difficult as headaches are for you to experience, witnessing a
headache attack can be just as upsetting to observers. They may be
frightened by your symptoms. They may be angered when you
miss activities. They may want to help you but don't know how. So
they may say or do things that aren't helpful or hesitate to discuss
concerns for fear they'll upset you.

You can help others help you by taking time to inform them
about your headaches and establishing open communication:

- Express your true feelings. Find appropriate ways to discuss concerns without attacking others. Even difficult emotions can be acknowledged in constructive ways.
- Ask for what you need. Don't expect others to know intuitively what's best for you. Be specific. Sometimes what you need is less attention focused on your headache or to be left alone when you have a headache.
- Discuss communication roadblocks. If communication between you and a friend becomes one-sided, consider how you can change that. If someone accuses you of using headaches as an excuse, try not to react defensively.
- Get help if you can't resolve problems. Counseling can help get you and your loved ones talking to each other.

Support groups

Headache support groups provide forums to discuss the various concerns of group members living with chronic or severe pain. Your participation in a support group can give you a depth of understanding that you might not find anywhere else. Group meetings put you face to face with people who have many of the same physical symptoms and emotional responses you do. Listening to other people's stories can reassure you that you're not the only one with these kinds of experiences. Sharing with others fosters an exchange of useful coping strategies.

Support groups aren't for everyone. You may feel hesitant about sharing your feelings with strangers. And if you're attending a group for the first time, it's OK if you choose not to speak up during the first sessions. Most groups have a facilitator who tries to help newcomers feel welcome and comfortable.

Look for a support group where the mood is upbeat and the message is positive. Some group meetings that aren't carefully monitored can become forums to vent only negative feelings. The facilitators should avoid "doctor bashing" and allow each person to share feelings and be treated respectfully.

Finding a support group. Your community may have one or more support groups for people with headaches or chronic pain. The American Council for Headache Education (ACHE) maintains a network of support groups across the country, as well as online support groups. If there's no ACHE support group in your area and you're interested in starting one, you can contact ACHE headquarters for more information.

Specialized therapy

Behavior therapy can be helpful for dealing with headaches, stress and the difficult emotions that often accompany headaches. You don't have to spend years in therapy or invest thousands of dollars in order to benefit from this form of treatment.

Using face-to-face interviews and discussions, a behavior therapist helps you understand the nature of your condition. More understanding can help you cope better with the circumstances of everyday living. The therapist uses techniques that help you change behavior that's not good for you and reinforce behavior that's helping you manage your headaches. This form of therapy is also an effective treatment for depression, anxiety and other mood disorders that affect many people with headaches.

If you choose to pursue behavior therapy, look for a therapist who is knowledgeable about your type of headache and understands that headaches are biological disorders — not psychological in origin. You may want to ask your primary doctor for a referral to a specialist.

When to seek professional help

You don't have to be in dire circumstances to benefit from specialized therapy. But extreme emotions may require more prompt action. Don't delay seeking professional guidance if:

- You have thoughts of suicide
- You lose interest in things you've always enjoyed doing, even when you're not having headaches
- You develop extreme fears that interrupt your normal moods, such as thinking your headaches are a sign of imminent death, or you avoid leaving the house for fear of having a headache

Maintaining your emotional balance

When headache pain disrupts your life, you may find yourself overwhelmed by a jumble of intense emotions:

Powerlessness. You can't predict when headaches occur, and the measures you take can't always prevent them.

Guilt. You feel like you're letting down those who depend on you. You may believe you bring the headaches on yourself.

Shame. You worry that headaches are a sign that you're weak or can't handle stress. You may sense that others are judging you.

Frustration. You think, why me? You've tried to control your headaches and nothing seems to work.

Depression. You're overwhelmed by feelings of worthlessness. You lose interest in favorite activities and can't concentrate.

Isolation. You feel that no one understands what you're going through and that others aren't sympathetic.

Don't feel ashamed if these emotions sometimes get the better of you. Living with headaches can be difficult. For many people, a positive first step is to acknowledge that these feelings exist. Over time, you'll learn to stop focusing on things you can't change, and, instead, look to the future. The following suggestions may help you work through your emotions:

- Recognize the serious impact of headaches on your life. Don't trivialize them.
- Give yourself time for an emotional adjustment. Living with headaches is not an excuse to be unkind or insensitive. But feelings of frustration, sadness and resentment are normal, and you deserve the time to work through them.
- Learn to say no to excessive demands when you have a headache coming on. Make your body's needs a priority.
- Treat yourself and others with respect. Nurture social contact — talk with a friend, attend an event, help someone else.
- Find creative ways to express what you're feeling. You might write in a journal, listen to music or pursue a hobby.

Practice positive thinking. Self-talk is the stream of thoughts that run through your head every day. Monitor your self-talk and try to replace negative thoughts with positive ones. Reduce stress and stay physically active. Stress management and exercise promote a general sense of well-being.

How you organize your day can affect how you manage your headaches. If you overwork or overcommit yourself, fatigue and frustration may set in, making it harder to handle headache symptoms. The opposite isn't better — avoiding daily activities and spending hours at home anticipating the next attack can isolate you and focus your attention only on your pain.

The best solution is a healthy balance of work, socialization, exercise and relaxation throughout the day. Achieving such a balance is tricky. Like many people, you may have a full schedule of commitments and responsibilities. Success will require you to plan, prioritize and delegate those responsibilities. Instead of making a sudden, drastic alteration to your routine, plan a series of small changes that you can incorporate one at a time.

Staying productive at home, work and school

Headaches can turn your day upside down. You begin the morning alert and energetic. Your schedule is busy but not overloaded. You plan on running several errands and continuing to work on that project you've started. You're looking forward to a relaxing evening with friends. Then, a headache starts.

At home
The strain of living with chronic headaches can take a heavy toll on your family. Time set aside for domestic duties and shared activities is often delayed or lost due to pain. Frequent attacks leave little time for sexual intimacy, while some headache medications may reduce sexual interest. The expense of medications and medical care can cause financial difficulties.

Headaches can also affect your ability to be an active parent. You may not be able to pick up the kids from school regularly, or you might miss important parent-child activities. The expense of extra child care adds to the financial burden. These problems can lead to conflicts with your spouse.

The following tips can help keep your home life on track:

- Make sure your spouse or partner is aware of the impact headaches have on your ability to function. Relate as much as you know about when the headaches come and how long they last. Also try to keep your children informed.
- Establish procedures that help your spouse or partner overcome your sudden absence in the midst of a busy day, such as getting meals ready or picking the kids up from school. Develop backup plans for many contingencies. This may include asking others to help out occasionally.
- Make sure your spouse or partner is comfortable performing tasks that you do routinely when you don't have a headache. At the same time, it's important not to deviate drastically from these routines when headaches are present.
- If current headache medications are affecting your interest in sex, talk to your doctor about changing medications or modifying your dosage. If you're having problems with sexual intimacy because of fear, worry or guilt about your headaches, you may want to consult a counselor to learn more constructive ways of handling these emotions.

At work

You may find it hard to balance the demands of your job with the demands of keeping your headache under control. Many people with frequent, severe headaches have trouble staying productive, let alone performing at peak efficiency, while at work. Some choose to hide their condition from their employer and stay on the job during all but the worst headache attacks. They fear asking for the support they need from co-workers.

Many employers are not particularly knowledgeable about chronic headaches. They may be more aware of headaches that are occasional and often resolved with over-the-counter pain relievers. With greater awareness, employers may benefit from offering flexible scheduling and other options to employees with chronic headaches. Studies show that, with these measures, a company can gain more in productivity, loyalty and job satisfaction than it can lose in sick time and insurance benefits.

If you're worried about informing an employer about your headaches, be aware that you do have legal protections. Under the Americans With Disabilities Act (ADA), employers can't discriminate against qualified people with disabilities, including chronic headaches, if the employee can perform the job with what's known as reasonable accommodation. A reasonable accommodation is any modification to job responsibilities or work environments that enables an employee with a disability to perform essential tasks.

If you choose to discuss your headaches with your employer, here are a couple of tips to help you:

- Address the issue openly and directly, and provide details about your headaches. Your employer needs to be fully aware of how they affect you.
- Offer practical suggestions that might reasonably accommodate your needs in the workplace. For example, if a strong odor such as perfume is a migraine trigger, suggest that headaches might be less frequent if you could work in a perfume-free environment.

If you're self-employed, you have more flexibility with your schedule and more control of your work environment. But self-employment has drawbacks as well. For one thing, if you can't work due to headaches, you don't earn income. Also, insurance for a self-employed individual can be prohibitively expensive.

At school

Children who get disabling headaches can be challenged to keep up with the demands of school. Depending on the severity of your child's headaches, some missed school days probably are inevitable. But most children with headaches can keep up with their schoolwork even if they miss some time. For those children who have headaches that don't respond well to treatment, frequent absences may threaten their academic progress. These children may need to participate in special programs for students who are homebound due to illness.

Headaches may take a tremendous emotional toll on your child, especially during those times when he or she wants to fit in and be like everyone else. Some children develop a phobia about going to school — they're afraid of having an attack in front of their peers. You may inadvertently reinforce your child's anxiety by keeping him or her out of school longer than necessary.

Here are some suggestions for helping children with headaches manage better at school:

- Inform teachers, school nurses and guidance counselors about your child's headaches and their impact on his or her life.
- Avoid keeping your child home from school more than necessary. Be firm but loving when confronting the child's fears of having a headache attack at school.
- Support your child's longings for a normal life by helping him or her gain a sense of control and motivation to succeed.

Setting goals

To gain control of your headaches, you need a workable plan. Should you strive to be completely headache-free, or is it better to aim for having only one headache a month? Perhaps you should try to eliminate headache triggers, or maintain a regular sleep schedule. The key to your plan is to set goals that are specific, measurable, attainable, realistic and trackable (SMART):

Specific. State exactly what you want to achieve, how you're going to do it and when you want to achieve it. It's often helpful to plan a series of small goals instead of one big, all-encompassing goal.

Measurable. Be sure you can tell whether you've achieved a goal or not. For example, if your goal is to walk for 30 minutes a day, you'll know when you've achieved it.

Attainable. Ask yourself whether a goal is within reasonable reach before you set it. Are you allowing sufficient time and resources? Start slowly and work your way up to larger goals.

Realistic. Set goals that are within your capabilities, and take into account your limitations. For example, a realistic goal might be to lower the frequency of headache attacks by 50 percent rather than eliminating them altogether.

Trackable. Recording your progress in a headache diary or exercise log helps keep you motivated.

Insurance issues

For many people, the health insurance system can be frustrating to navigate. The U. S. health care market is complex, and many consumers struggle to find adequate coverage, deal with a myriad of insurance companies and managed care companies, and cover the high cost of medications.

Health care costs add up quickly if your condition is chronic. Some people with chronic headaches pay for medical care through either their health insurance carriers or government programs such as Medicare and Medicaid. Others lack health insurance entirely or buy catastrophic insurance only, paying for most medications and treatments out of their own pockets.

In the United States, more than half the population receives health care through managed care systems such as HMO's (health maintenance organizations). With a managed care plan, the insurer or HMO signs contracts with certain doctors and hospitals (often called providers) to care for plan members. Your primary care doctor usually serves as the gatekeeper who refers you to specialists when necessary. For example, if you have severe migraine, your doctor, who may be a family physician, may refer you to a headache specialist.

Some people with chronic headaches have no problem getting adequate health insurance coverage for their treatments. Others must invest time and energy to appeal coverage claims that have been denied. For example, being reimbursed for a headache-related diagnosis can be difficult sometimes because there's no laboratory test or other diagnostic marker for headaches. Health insurers may question a doctor's evaluation and recommended treatment for headaches. Some health plans refuse to pay for any nonmedication therapies. When you start a new job, the new insurer may not cover pre-existing medical conditions, such as chronic headaches, for a specified period of time, for example, 12 months.

Understanding your health plan
Your best bet for getting the best possible outcome from the health care system is to be informed about your health plan's coverage, as

well as your own medical condition. Take the time to read your insurance policy. If you have questions about coverage, ask a company representative to explain it. Be sure that you're knowledgeable about the following issues in your health plan:

- Coverage of acute and preventive medical care
- Guidelines for seeing specialists
- Guidelines for getting special services or tests
- Prescription drug benefits
- Coverage of chronic illnesses

Most managed care plans have a list of approved prescription medicines, called a drug formulary. If a drug you need isn't on the formulary, you'll probably have to pay more for it. In some plans, your doctor can request authorization for a drug that's not on the list. Review the formulary, and ask if your plan allows for a doctor's authorization.

Most health plans provide full coverage for the management of many chronic illnesses, but some headache therapies may not be covered. If your doctor decides you need to have surgery or have certain tests done, your insurer may require pre-authorization (preapproval) of the treatment.

Here are other tips for handling insurance issues:

- Be aware that your insurance company, not your doctor, makes decisions about what will be paid for and what won't be. Your doctor might be familiar with your coverage, but he or she may not know the specific details.
- If your insurance company denies a claim, you have the right to appeal, or challenge, the decision. The appeal process should be explained in your health plan's handbook. If your doctor agrees that you should make an appeal, he or she may be able to help you through the process.
- If your insurance company refuses to pay your claim after an appeal, or drops you from your plan, consider contacting your state's insurance commissioner.
- Don't let your policy lapse, and pay your premiums on time. If you plan to change jobs, find out if your insurance will transfer. If you must switch to a different insurer, check if the new plan will cover your pre-existing condition.

- If your primary care doctor seems uninterested in taking care of chronic headaches, you have the right to choose a new doctor from your managed care plan's list of providers.
- Don't put off critical medical care because of cost. If insurance coverage is a problem, talk with your doctor or the clinic administrator. They may be able to suggest alternative ways to cover the cost.
- Be persistent about seeing a specialist if standard headache treatments aren't working. Many managed care plans will refer you to someone outside the network if you make a good case for it.

Staying positive

A positive perspective is vital to managing your headaches. If you are committed to living a full, satisfying life whether or not you have headaches, you've armed yourself with one of the most important components of success — hope.

No doubt, you'll have difficult days. You'll have times when pain gets the best of you. To help stay in control of your headaches, regularly use the strategies outlined in this book, such as exercise, relaxation and the appropriate use of medications.

And give yourself credit for what you've accomplished. It takes courage and strength to face chronic bouts of pain and the disruption that results from severe headaches. Acknowledge the hard work you've put into making your life better.

Additional resources

American Council for Headache Education

19 Mantua Road
Mt. Royal, NJ 08061
(856) 423-0258
www.achenet.org

American Headache Society

19 Mantua Road
Mount Royal, NJ 08061
(856) 423-0043
www.ahsnet.org

International Headache Society

9 Willowmead Drive
Prestbury, Cheshire
SK10 4BU
United Kingdom
44 1625 828663
www.i-h-s.org

Mayo Clinic Health Information

www.MayoClinic.com

Migraine Awareness Group: A National Understanding for Migraineurs (MAGNUM)

113 S. Saint Asaph, Suite 300
Alexandria, VA 22314
(703) 739-9384
www.migraines.org

National Headache Foundation

820 N. Orleans St., Suite 217
Chicago, IL 60610
(888) 643-5552
www.headaches.org

Trigeminal Neuralgia Association

2801 S.W. Archer Road
Gainesville, FL 32608
(352) 376-9955
www.tna-support.org

World Headache Alliance

3288 Old Coach Road
Burlington, Ontario
Canada L7N 3P7
www.w-h-a.org

Associated organizations

American Academy of Orofacial Pain

19 Mantua Road
Mount Royal, NJ 08061
(856) 423-3629
www.aaop.org

American Academy of Pain Medicine

4700 W. Lake Avenue
Glenview, IL 60025
(847) 375-4731
www.painmed.org

American Chronic Pain Association

P.O. Box 850
Rocklin, CA 95677
(800) 533-3231
www.theacpa.org

American Neurological Association
5741 Cedar Lake Road, Suite 204
Minneapolis, MN 55416
(952) 545-6284
www.aneuroa.org

American Pain Foundation
201 N. Charles St., Suite 710
Baltimore, MD 21201-4111
(888) 615-7246
www.painfoundation.org

American Pain Society
4700 W. Lake Ave.
Glenview, IL 60025
(847) 375-4715
www.ampainsoc.org

Brain Aneurysm Foundation
12 Clarendon St.
Boston, MA 02116
(617) 723-3870
www.bafound.org

Brain Injury Association of America
8201 Greensboro Drive, Suite 611
McLean, VA 22102
(703) 761-0750 or (800) 444-6443
www.biausa.org

International Association for the Study of Pain
909 N.E. 43d Street, Suite 306
Seattle, WA 98105
(206) 547-6409
www.iasp-pain.org

Meningitis Foundation of America

6610 N. Shadeland Ave., Suite 200
Indianapolis, IN 46220-4393
(800) 668-1129
www.musa.org

National Brain Tumor Foundation

414 13th St., Suite 700
Oakland, CA 94612-2603
(510) 839-9777 or (800) 934-2873
www.braintumor.org

National Center for Complementary and Alternative Medicine

P.O. Box 7923
Gaithersburg, MD 20898
(888) 644-6226
www.nccam.nih.gov

National Foundation for the Treatment of Pain

P.O. Box 70045
Houston, TX 77270-0045
(713) 862-9332
www.paincare.org

National Institute of Neurological Disorders and Stroke

P. O. Box 5801
Bethesda, MD 20824
(800) 352-9424
http://accessible.ninds.nih.gov/index.html

National Pain Foundation

3511 S. Clarkson Street
Denver, CO 80113
(303) 756-0889
www.painconnection.org

Glossary

abdominal migraine. Form of migraine occurring primarily in children, characterized by pain in the abdomen rather than in the head and accompanied by nausea and vomiting.

acute. Term to describe a headache that is severe and lasts a short time. The onset may be sudden. Acute treatment is taken to diminish or stop headache symptoms such as pain and nausea once an attack has started.

analgesic. Pain reliever, generally over the counter, that's often the first line of treatment for mild to moderately severe headaches.

antiemetic. Drug that may relieve the nausea and vomiting often associated with migraine.

aura. Neurological symptoms that come before, and sometimes accompany, migraine pain. These symptoms include blind spots and flashing lights in your visual field, numbness or tingling sensations, and muscular weakness.

autonomic nervous system. Portion of the nervous system that controls many life-sustaining activities without your consciously having to think about and regulate them, for example, blood pressure, heartbeat, sweating and body temperature.

basilar-type migraine. Form of migraine with aura that originates at the brainstem, causing temporary blindness and other possible symptoms.

bilateral headache. Headache with pain occurring on both sides of the head.

brain abscess. Mass made up of immune cells, pus and other materials that develops from a brain infection.

brain tumor. Abnormal mass of cells that grow in the brain, which can be a relatively rare cause of headache.

butalbital. Sedative drug (barbituate) that's sometimes included with an analgesic to form an effective combination drug for headache.

cephalalgia. Another word for headache, originating from an ancient Greek word meaning "head pain."

cerebral aneurysm. Condition that occurs when a weakened blood vessel wall bulges under the pressure of circulating blood. A burst aneurysm leads to subarachnoid hemorrhage and headache.

chronic. Term to describe headaches that occur frequently over a long period of time.

chronic daily headache. Designation for several different types of headaches that share a common characteristic of occurring several hours a day nearly every day.

cluster headache. Type of primary headache characterized by severe pain in and around one eye, a teary eye and stuffy nose. Multiple attacks occur in cyclical patterns or "clusters."

confusional migraine. Form of migraine with aura that affects the centers of consciousness in your brain, resulting in problems with concentration and difficulty with speech and motor skills.

dissection. Condition in which blood leaks into an artery wall and collects there, forming a clot that may block blood flow.

dura mater. Outermost layer of the meninges that covers and protects the brain.

encephalitis. Inflammation of the brain usually caused by a viral infection.

episodic. Term to describe a headache that is a separate event but still forming part of a larger series — meaning each headache has a definite beginning and ending separated by discrete periods of time before the next attack.

hemicrania continua. Type of chronic daily headache characterized by pain on one side of the head only.

hemiplegic migraine. Form of migraine accompanied by stroke-like symptoms with paralysis on one side of the body and, usually, other neurological symptoms.

hemorrhagic stroke. Form of stroke in which an artery in the brain ruptures, leaking blood into the brain and causing brain cell damage.

hydrocephalus. Emergency complication caused by a blockage of cerebrospinal fluid, which builds up in and around the brain.

hypnic headache. Moderate to severe headache that develops at night, occurring primarily among older adults.

hypothalamus. Portion of the brain that controls the sleep-wake cycle and other internal rhythms. It's thought to play a role in cluster headache development.

intracranial hypotension. Abnormally low pressure of the cerebrospinal fluid.

ischemic stroke. Form of stroke in which blood supply to the brain is blocked, damaging brain cells. A transient ischemic attack (TIA) sometimes is called a mini-stroke or stroke warning because the temporary disruption of blood flow increases your risk of a full ischemic stroke.

lumbar puncture. Procedure, also called a spinal tap, that's used to test and to relieve the pressure of cerebrospinal fluid.

meninges. Three layers of membrane that envelop and protect the brain.

meningitis. Inflammation of the membranes and fluid surrounding the brain and spinal cord caused by a bacterial, viral or fungal infection.

menstrually-associated migraine. Form of migraine in which attacks occur throughout the monthly cycle but increase in frequency or intensity at the time of your period.

migraine. Type of primary headache characterized by moderate to severe pain and often accompanied by nausea and sensitivity to light and sound. Migraine may be preceded by aura.

neurotransmitter. Chemical in the brain that transmits electric impulses, allowing nerves to communicate.

new daily persistent headache. Type of chronic daily headache that often has an abrupt onset in people who have had no history of frequent headaches.

nociceptor. Nerve ending that can detect stimuli, such as a cut, burn or inflammation, and relay pain messages to the brain.

nonvascular intracranial disorder. Disorder within the skull that is unrelated to problems with the cerebral blood vessels.

phonophobia. Extreme sensitivity to noise.

photophobia. Extreme sensitivity to light.

postheadache phase. Final phase of a migraine attack, in which all headache symptoms disappear.

postherpetic neuralgia. Form of neuralgia that generally occurs in older adults as a complication of shingles, when the chickenpox virus is reactivated inside your nerve cells.

premonitory phase. Initial phase of a migraine when certain signs and symptoms indicate a headache is coming on, including depression, weakness, difficulty with concentration and stiff neck. This phase, also called the prodrome, is not the same as the aura.

preventive treatment. Headache treatment taken to stop headaches from happening. It also may reduce the duration of an attack or diminish the intensity of pain when headaches occur.

primary headache. Headache that isn't caused by an underlying condition. There's no clear source for the pain.

pure menstrual migraine. Form of migraine in which attacks occur regularly around the onset of a period and at no other time during the menstrual cycle.

rebound headache. Also known as medication-induced headache, which results from the overuse of headache medications.

secondary headache. Headache that is a symptom of another disease or condition.

serotonin. Brain chemical (see *neurotransmitter*) that regulates pain messages and is believed to be a factor in headaches.

sinusitis. Condition in which sinus membranes become swollen and inflamed, trapping mucus in the air-filled cavities.

status migrainosus. Complication of migraine, characterized by severe pain and nausea lasting for more than 72 hours.

subarachnoid hemorrhage. Condition caused by blood leaking into the brain and spinal fluid from a ruptured aneurysm.

subdural hematoma. Condition caused by blood collecting beneath the outer covering of the brain (dura mater), often following head trauma.

temporomandibular joint (TMJ). Hinge joint located on each side of your head that connects the lower jawbone to your skull.

tension-type headache. Type of primary headache characterized by mild to moderate, dull, aching pain that's often described as a band of pressure around the head.

thalamus. Structure in your brain that serves as a clearinghouse for information, such as incoming pain messages, that needs to be relayed to other parts of the brain.

trigeminal autonomic cephalalgia (TAC). Designation for several different headaches, including cluster headache, characterized by stabbing pain and a response from the autonomic nervous system.

trigeminal nerve. One of the 12 cranial nerve pairs in your head and a major pathway to your brain for sensory information from all areas of your face.

trigeminal neuralgia. Sudden, short bursts of severe facial pain that result from the abnormal function of the trigeminal nerve.

trigger. External or internal factors that may contribute to the onset of a headache. Many people find that their headaches occur in response to a specific trigger – for example, something they ate, a strong odor, a change in the weather or a stressful environment.

triptan. Drug developed to relieve migraine symptoms such as pain and nausea. For people with severe attacks, triptans are often the drug of choice.

unilateral headache. Headache with pain occurring on only one side of the head.

Index